The Faeries' Guide to Green Magick from the Garden

The Faeries' Guide to Green Magick from the Garden

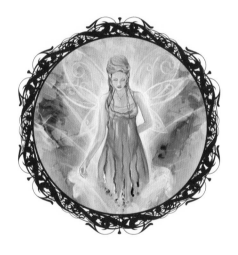

Jamie Wood and Lisa Steinke

Illustrations by Lisa Steinke

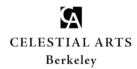

CELESTIAL ARTS

Berkeley

I dedicate this book to the fae whom I refer to as nature shamans, and whose essence is the guiding force, power, and beauty of all things wild.

—Jamie Wood

Dedicated to my family who keeps the magick alive in my heart, and to Robert Gould who keeps the magick alive in my art.

—Lisa Steinke

Published in the United States by Celestial Arts, a division of Ten Speed Press, an imprint of the Crown Publishing Group, a division of Random House, Inc., New York.
www.crownpublishing.com
www.tenspeed.com

Celestial Arts and the Celestial Arts colophon are registered trademarks of Random House, Inc.

Library of Congress Cataloging-in-Publication Data
Wood, Jamie.
  The faeries' guide to green magick from the garden / Jamie Wood ;
illustrated by Lisa Steinke. — 1st ed.
    p. cm.
  Includes index.
  1. Magic. 2. Gardening—Miscellanea.
  3. Herbs—Miscellanea. 4. Recipes.
  5. Fairies. I. Title.

  BF1623.G37W66 2010
  133'.258163—dc22

2010002824

ISBN 978-1-58761-354-8
First Edition

Printed in China

Design by Chloe Rawlins

10 9 8 7 6 5 4 3 2 1

Contents

An Invitation

There is a place
Between here and there,
Between us and them.
Below the stars,
Above the noise,
Within the silence.
A place of connection for all living things,
of wonder and discovery.
Wander in and take a peek
For you have been invited,
And we have been waiting for you.

The Faeries' Guide to Green Magick

Throughout time, people of every society have turned to the earth and attuned themselves to the web of life that pulses through all living things and found the means to sustain themselves. Whether they sought comfort from lavender or mending a broken bone with comfrey, ancient people knew that the way to ensure their health, survival, and security was to call upon the rich supply of the earth's herbs, plants, and trees.

And yet, our ancestors did not stop at the point of just receiving. They developed and carefully cultivated a symbiotic, give-and-take, stewardship with the earth. They tended to the healing and nourishing of plant life as tenderly as they took care of their own children, all the while understanding it was they who were dependent upon the earth and not the other way around. Their humility helped them forge a reverential relationship with the life force that vibrated within each plant and tree. And by tapping into the earth's pulsing life, they were part of the green magick that expanded the positive energy and vitality of the earth itself, which in turn increased the health of humans, animals, insects, and all plant life.

As we carelessly and often unconsciously, deplete the earth's resources, we have lost touch with the magick that was once at our fingertips. Many look aside as wild, verdant lands, and animal and plant species essential to the delicate balance of life, disappear at an alarming rate. By distancing from nature, we have essentially denied ourselves the connection that would bring wholeness, abundance, and peace to our lives. In fact, our innate ability to heal ourselves has become a nearly lost art. When we forgot the heart of nature is our own heart, we created a way of life that taxes the earth's precious resources and created the need to manufacture what was once organic and easily available. The result has created fierce competition, fear of dominance, and overwhelming feelings of lack.

Ask yourself, when did nature become something to avoid, and why? We are nature, like a giraffe, a butterfly, a river, lichen, or chamomile. We just need to remember. We need to piece ourselves back together by reestablishing our connection to the earth. We need to reclaim the magick of our bond with the life force that unites us all. There has been no other time in the age of humanity in which the importance of cultivating an ongoing relationship with Mother Earth has taken on such vital importance. This back-to-nature perspective, today's green movement, is at once practical and spiritual, as everyday life used to be.

Being eco-friendly is much more than buying halogen lightbulbs or using cloth bags. It means we once again form a friendship with our ecosystem. This is no ordinary friendship, but a sacred relationship with the life force teeming through plants, herbs, and trees. This life force—the sentient energy that exists at the heart of each plant—is the *faerie* or *deva* of each plant. The synergy of our sacred relationship with this energy is the green magick, the healing serendipity, and the wonder found when we develop a bond with nature. When we truly understand, recognize, and believe in the living soul within each being, within fauna *and* flora, one by one our collective compassion awakens and it becomes essential to preserve and protect the earth—our home.

When you draw from botanical resources, whether you are flavoring food or working with essential oils for healing, you are tapping into an intelligent life force.

When you cultivate a garden you are tending to a living being, whose response to your attention is seen in its growth pattern and increased potency in your recipes. The more you become aware of the consciousness of the botanical realm and the deeper your respect of the life in each plant, the better cook, healer, or gardener you will become because the plants give you an exact exchange for the energy you give them. Your acknowledgment of the plant's true essence helps carry the highest potentiality into every concoction you will make. The time has come to develop a culture of interconnection and communion with the earth energy—the faeries.

Each faerie has an individual personality, which can appear as a reflection of the plant, tree, or natural element where it resides. Fae or devic energy can also take on abstract forms, such as a blanket of color or the oscillating energy of heat rising from asphalt in hundred-degree weather. Fae can appear as a chorus of winged creatures or as a beautiful woman or man. It may shift from an individual to a collective form and back again. Most certainly, faeries will shake up whatever you thought you knew about them. Consider how long plants have been around. Their intelligence far exceeds our own, and so it is to them that we turn for healing.

The unique expression of each fae as captured by the text and paintings in this book speaks to the intrinsic qualities, traits, and behavior of each herb or tree. Faeries are beings in and of themselves, as humans are beings. Faeries are a separate race, coexisting alongside us, like the birds bringing food to their young or the bees pollinating the flowers as you walk to work. The images of faerie essences found in this book will bring us closer to their feeling rather than their form. The paintings of our faeries are an experiential interpretation of the faerie, or life force energy, of each herb or tree. The images represent sensation, as if you could put a picture to the taste that bounces around in your mouth when you eat an herb or smell a flower. When you give faeries the respect and acknowledgment as the living essence of plant life, whole new vistas of possibilities open up for you, and then the true magick can begin.

Magick spelled with a "k" differentiates the word from "magic," as in tricks performed for entertainment. It also represents the realm of possibilities, *expected* serendipity, connection to all living things, and a deep reverence and wonder for nature. The spelling is symbolic and carries deep meaning, pointing directly to the vibrant intersection of where heaven meets earth. The "g" points to the ground or form, similar to a vortex triangle that points to the earth and is generally yin, female, or resting energy. The "k" reaches for the sky, where ideas are born, similar to the upward-pointing apex triangle that is typically considered yang, and represents the male, or active energy.

The overlapping vortex and apex triangles create a symbol, often known as the Star of David. The intersection of form and thought is where magick happens. The connection represents the material and the spiritual coming together to develop the soul. In magickal circles, we refer to this concept with the phrase "As above, so below." The soul's work on earth is not complete if it dwells too long in the spiritual realm or mundane reality. It must unite male and female, light and dark, intangible and material, heaven and earth to create magick. On earth, we live in that powerful meeting place where form is created from desire and need.

The four elements of nature are the fundamental tools of magick. Humans are a representation of the four elements working in sync: *earth* is our bodies, *water* is our blood, *air* is our breath, and *fire* is our energy or spirit. Magick is that feeling when events and people in our life line up with ease and enlightened intention. When you get that tingly sensation and the air feels thick with electricity, you are in the infinite realm of illimitable potential—the womb of creation.

Magickal spells are a matter of aligning your desire with symbolic interpretations of what you want to create (for example, a collage board), then speaking aloud your intention. The etymology of the word *spell* means "to cast or speak your word." It is no different than a prayer. Rhymes found in spells speak to the right brain, the part of our consciousness that is most like the cyclical dreamtime world, when anything is possible. Spells are used to change circumstances. Rituals, such as a ceremony to let go of anger or achieve forgiveness, are used to change consciousness.

Tuning in to nature and herbs can help bring the spiritual to the mundane, heaven to earth. Sit with your plants. Visualize the energy that lives in each little herb. Whatever reveals itself to you, is perfect for you. Recognize that you are cultivating friendship with another being. There is no right or wrong way to see the faeries.

Developing a relationship with a singular herb was how the shamans and ancient healers approached unknown plants so many hundreds of years ago. They would meditate with the plants and ask for an interpretation of what the plants had to offer. The message might come in a dream, arise as a symbol, or present itself when a patient was in need. How else could they have determined that inside the spiny leaves of the aloe was a soothing gel that would bring relief to a burn? The plants are just as eager to develop a relationship with you as you are excited to begin working with them. As we become more "green," we begin to fulfill our destiny to live in harmony, symbiosis, and balance with nature.

The call to reduce our carbon footprints essentially points to the fact that we must stop taking up so much space and give room for the plants to grow. And as we create balance, we discover that every living creature needs water, food, shelter, and space to survive. What can be more important than allowing space for the plant *kin-dom* that provides us with food and medicine?

One of the most important things to remember as you join or deepen your experience in green magick is to begin the process in a way that is comfortable to you. You don't need to get overwhelmed by the long list of eco-friendly advice. Feeling guilt or pressure will not help you develop a healthy relationship with the earth spirits. You must begin, yes, but allow each step toward becoming green to ease itself into your lifestyle. Start by talking with your plants, shop at farmers' markets, plant an herb or veggie garden, even if it's just in pots on your balcony. There is no judgment on this path back to trusting and taking care of Mother Earth.

By harkening back to the times of our ancestors, we will embrace nature once again and the magick will return to our lives. No matter how refined or sophisticated we may pretend to be, deep down we miss the magick. In magick there is wonder, appreciation, and security. Although we may have attempted to take what gifts the earth has provided for us and "improve" upon them, the faerie spirit continues to press its way into our lives, crying out for us to stop fixing what was never broken. And at long last, we begin to take a look at ourselves and the treasures around us.

The faeries have not forgotten our true nature. As we begin to relate more deeply to the living essence of the earth, we will nurture our own planet back to health. The earth and all that grows on her will respond with vibrant aliveness to our attention, and a meaningful, abundant, reciprocal relationship will develop. As you develop your unique relationship with the faeries, you will discover that the magick is simply there and the faeries surround you.

What Is Faerie?

"Faeries are the inner nature of the land and
a reflection of the inner nature of our souls."
—Brian Froud, *Good Faeries / Bad Faeries*

Faerie energy is the *prana* of the earth, the life source, intelligence, and breath of the plants. It is the essence of the life in nature. Fae energy is the family of the many diverse types of essence or spirit in all of nature. Dryads are found in trees. Naiads are the energy of the rivers and streams. Gnomes live in hills and mountains and under the earth. Sylphs float in the air. Faeries live in plants, herbs, and flowers. They all live in another dimension from our material form, although they coexist with humans in the spiritual, emotional, and mental planes.

Faeries are free from dense form, unless they choose to assume a shape. Faeries are a reflection of the natural vessels that contain them and take on the aspects of the plant, whether through the physicality of the plant or herb, the etymology of its name, or the healing or magickal properties of the plant.

Formlessness has been an obstacle for the understanding of faerie energy underlined by the saying "Seeing is believing." In an effort to connect with human friends, faeries will take on an outward appearance that can be best understood and received by the human whose attention they are seeking. The exception would be if they intend to help you evolve beyond a narrow vision to something broader. Our egocentrism and fear of the unknown is why so many people are drawn to faerie images in which these feral, elemental creatures look like beautiful humans.

Try experimenting with a group of people and sit with an herb. Have everyone close their eyes and meditate on the life force of the plant. The group may end up with very different interpretations, which is similar to when different people look at the same situation but come away with different perspectives based on their beliefs, position in the room, and expectations. You might discover that several people have the same vision of the plant's life force. This result is an example of people tapping into the collective consciousness, a cloud of energy floating above—as if they are tuned in to the same radio station. A common example of this occurrence is when you are thinking of a song and someone standing next to you begins to sing the song aloud.

Essentially, a faerie's deepest expression is as the breath, intelligence, and life force of Mother Earth. Our vision of a humanlike faerie is an attempt to understand by creating something visually familiar. And yet, we believe in love, though we cannot see it. We are beginning to understand through quantum physics that our attention largely affects what we see. We are beginning to disengage from defining the image and releasing expectations. We are beginning to allow the essences or spirits of the fae to reveal themselves to us on their own terms.

Faerie is the energy that grants you permission to be free. Faerie is the spirit that moves you beyond restrictions and guidelines. It bursts through condemnation and fear. It is the confidence that grants you protection from others' opinions and judgments. Faerie energy allows you to fly, to reach for your dreams. Faerie is the energy and impulse that leads you to your true self.

Faeries can be amoral, impish, light, or dark. Fae can be playful, but because faeries feel nothing of societal criticism or disapproval, fae energy can drive you straight to a whole mess of drama, without the slightest feeling of remorse. In fact, some say that your drama is their entertainment. Fae don't take themselves as seriously as humans tend to do. In the faerie realm, fear is nothing more than a test of trust. Think of all the exciting energy derived from trouble—it's quite a visceral, magickal feeling, with a lot of potential for growth and a fresh new perspective. Faeries' version of play often produces chaos—from which we create. Faeries simply love to see the expansion of life.

Many faeries desire to aid and bring human friends good fortune. Other faeries prefer to introduce the shadow side of life, which can be equally as helpful. In order to assist humans, faeries must be asked. Faeries delight in the attention and will be more helpful the more they receive considerate interest from you. Your attention determines the amount of energy they lend to you.

Faerie energy implores us to reach beyond the confining limitations of form, to feel and acknowledge energy in its essence, whether that be hope, love, or happiness. When you befriend and connect with the essence of a faerie, with the internal core, rather than focus on the external expression of the spirit, you will be better able to access the plant's healing and magickal properties. Focus your attention on the fae's formlessness and you will discover true magick. Draw your awareness to the fae energy as feeling, intelligent beings and their particular healing and magickal energy becomes integrated into you. With this deeper relationship you will tap into a reservoir of vitality, freedom, trust, healing, and fertile abundance—the core of the Mother-Father tantric dance of creation. All this and more is waiting for you as you enter the faerie realm.

Green Gardening

Every living being has intelligence and a predisposition to seek and sustain life. Just think of the plants that reach for the sun or the roots that reach for the good rich dirt. There could be no creature who would want the return of a pure, chemical-free earth more than the faeries themselves. Faeries support life and living in harmony and synergy with the earth and her creatures. The green movement concepts such as localization of food sources, seasonal peak food consumption, permaculture, xeriscape, composting, and companion planting are intrinsically supported by faeries.

Allow the process of becoming green to unfold naturally, organically, just like a magickal garden reveals itself slowly. You can simply practice one technique until it becomes a way of life before integrating another form of green gardening. Or perhaps you will only stick with one method. Alternatively, you can support any one of these movements through charitable contributions, voting in support of their efforts, buying books and magazines on the subjects, or simply talking about it and creating awareness in your community.

Localization means that you buy food and herbs that are grown locally. Shopping at local farmers' markets, planting your own garden, or contributing time and energy to a community garden reduces packaging, natural resources spent on transportation, and pollution. In some cases, it could also lessen overharvesting and elimination of animal habitats. In addition, food grown locally has within it the energy that has naturally adapted to your environment and provides the nourishment needed for ailments associated with specific climates. Current research has proven that food grown in a naturally stressful environment contains adaptogens that help alleviate stress. And an old adage states that whatever plant or tree will bring you healing will grow naturally within twenty miles of where you live.

Eating foods at their seasonal peak will ensure that you draw upon the herbs or foods when they are most potent. It is akin to athletes performing at their prime age, agility, and strength. It's plainly logical to access the life force at the height of its effectiveness. It is also believed that eating seasonally can help reduce allergies. By purchasing local foods in season, you eliminate the environmental damage caused by shipping foods thousands of miles, your food dollar goes directly to the farmer, and your family will be able to enjoy the health benefits of eating fresh, unprocessed fruits and vegetables. Buying seasonal produce also provides an exciting opportunity to try new foods and to experiment with seasonal recipes. Perhaps most important, you feel better because you have increased your own vibrancy and energy levels with alive herbs and foods.

In spring, focus on tender, leafy vegetation, such as fresh parsley, nettles, and basil. In summer, stick with light, cooling herbs, such as peppermint and aloe. In fall, turn toward the more warming spices, such as ginger and comfrey. In winter, turn even more exclusively toward warming herbs, such as garlic and valerian.

The word *permaculture* is a blending of the words *permanent* and *agriculture*, as well as *permanent* and *culture*. Modern permaculture is a way of looking at a whole system, observing how the parts relate, and using long-term, sustainable working methods. The core values of permaculture are 1) acknowledging the earth is our home and the source of all life, 2) living as a community member of the earth, not apart from it, 3) supporting and helping all living things to develop healthy societies, and 4) living by the concept of *fair share*, which includes placing limits on consumption to ensure that earth's resources are used in ways that are fair to all involved. All of these values return us once again to creating a harmonic relationship with nature and the vibrant force in all living things.

Creating well-designed landscapes that conserve water while celebrating the beauty of native, drought-resistant species is called *xeriscaping*. Plant herbs and trees innately adapted to the soil, temperature, and climate of your area. Plants with similar water needs should be grouped together. This is a good practice for those of us who forget to water frequently or are highly sensitive to the need to conserve water.

Composting reduces the need to use chemical fertilizers that can seep toxic waste containing lead, cadium, mercury, arsenic, and dioxin into the soil and groundwater, endangering the entire ecosystem. Composting can be a simple process of throwing small scraps of vegetables and fruits, crushed eggshells, or coffee grounds onto your garden. Or composting can involve more complex methods. You can use a composting tumbler or create your own compost from wood boxes. I once used my kids' forgotten sandbox. It was a handmade wooden box about 6 feet by 10 feet and only 1 foot deep, which made it really easy to turn. I bought a large sheet of plywood to cover it and reduce flies. Within a couple of months I had what gardeners call "black gold" filled with worms and all manner of dark, musty dirt for my happy trees and plants.

A middle-of-the-road compost process, called "sheet composting" begins with turning the garden soil. Add 6 inches of organic mulch (such as straw or even newspaper), then a layer of yard waste, vegetable and fruit scraps, hair and nail clippings, ashes from the fireplace, eggshells, nutshells, and coffee grounds. Water on occasion, depending on the weather and how much green material you add. Compost should be moist, but not wet, kind of like a good cake. Turn your compost over every once in a while. Add soil, green material, and mulch as you go along. Soon enough, your soil will begin to heat up and literally cook to the consistency of crumbly charcoal, breaking down complex chemicals, killing off most plant diseases and harmful insects, and rendering the earth soluble again.

Many gardeners plant herbs that will specifically help a compost pile. Red clover supplies the earth with nitrogen. Dandelion adds copper to your compost and will double the iron. Yarrow gives copper, phosphates, and potash to the soil. Roman chamomile provides calcium. Eucalyptus leaves can deter insects. Comfrey leaves are high in minerals.

Companion planting means that you plant herbs and trees together that naturally assist one another, such as planting garlic near roses, which helps get rid of aphids. You can also use gray water with roses or other plants that need help with reducing aphids. Chamomile is helpful in the garden because it brings health to other plants and repels insects.

Green gardening can also affect your electric or gas bill. Try planting deciduous trees (trees that lose their leaves in the winter) on the south and east sides of your home. During hot summer months, leafy green trees block the sun and provide valuable shade that will help keep your home cool. When the trees are bare in the winter, the sun's rays will help heat your home, while providing a natural barrier against cold winds. Weed management can be handled by pouring scalding water onto the unwanted plant or adding a little white vinegar, a pinch of salt, or liquid dish soap to the water.

Magickal Gardening

Magickal gardening takes green gardening a step further by taking into consideration how the moon and other planetary cycles affect growing patterns and fruit production. There are two forms of magickal gardening that will deepen your connection to the faeries: lunar gardening and biodynamic gardening. Lunar gardening has been in practice since the Middle Ages and is based on the cycles of the moon. When the moon waxes (increases) or wanes (decreases) it pulls on the moisture in the soil just as it pulls on the water of the oceans, creating tides.

There are four phases of the moon that correspond to distinct gardening patterns. During the new or dark moon, it is the time to plant and transplant above-ground annuals that produce seeds outside the fruit, such as lettuce, spinach, celery, broccoli, cabbage, cauliflower, and grain crops. During this time, leaf and root growth are balanced. As the moon grows, waxing into its second phase, the time has come to clip herbs for increased growth, harvest root crops, and plant and transplant above-ground annuals that form seeds inside the fruit, such as beans, melons, peas, peppers, squash, and tomatoes (this is also a good time to cut your hair for good growth). When the moon is full, roots experience the most growth. Now is the time to plant slow-germinating seeds, as well as bulbs, biennials, perennials, and root crops. Take indoor plants outside to bathe in the full moonlight. As the moon wanes, harvest plants for storage and drying; prune, cultivate, and sow plants that require a strong root system, and weed.

The astrological sign the moon is passing through also affects the garden. In general, flowers prefer the moon's transit through air signs, most plants will thrive as the moon passes through water signs, harvest and weed during the fire signs, and earth signs are good for root crops.

Biodynamic gardening is based on the practice of maintaining the vitality of the earth's spirit. Rudolf Steiner, a philosopher, an educator, an agricultural expert, and a clairvoyant who lived during the turn of the twentieth century, offered the basic theories of this gardening technique. According to biodynamic gardening, soil, like the earth itself, is a living, breathing organism with a complex, interdependent cyclical system of growth, fruition, death, decay, and renewal. Maintaining balanced and healthy soil is obtained through observation, which is the key to biodynamic gardening principles. The movement of the stars, weather patterns, animal reactions, and plant growth are carefully recorded and assessed to determine how to best support the life force of the plant. Through continual observation and study of the various changing environments and conditions, we begin to grasp what is essential for each individual plant.

Biodynamic principles can be applied at any time in a plant's life. This philosophy shows you how to cocreate with the Divine by giving you tools to read the book of nature, which reveals itself slowly to you. With time, experience, and an open heart, you will learn how the sun, wind, water, and soil affect your garden and in what measure they support the life force of your individual plants. Words will appear on the pages of your nature book and will be written on your heart and soul. And you and the faeries will create a world of harmony and interdependence like a painter creates worlds on a canvas.

With careful attention to how the elements affect the plants, clear thought, and ever-present awareness of the earth's prana, biodynamic gardening offers a guide to attune ourselves once again to the life force we refer to as the faerie. By paying close attention, we can hope to understand the language of the elements, hear the voice of the earth spirit, and regain ancient wisdom and interconnection.

Lastly, magickal gardening includes simply talking to your plants. Close your eyes and see whether you can feel the energy of the plant. Remember that the fae can take on any shape, so don't be surprised or second-guess your intuition when you feel or sense their presence. You may choose to sing to the plants. Trace the outline of the plant with your finger or on a piece of paper and allow your song to dip and soar with the herb's silhouette.

When planting herbs, be sure to massage the roots and moisten the soil before you plant them. To be certain you are tapping into the highest life force from the herbs, harvest after the roots have fully developed, during the peak of their growth, and in the morning after the dew has evaporated. Harvest the fresh leaves below the flowers, but do not take insect-bitten, yellowed, or blotched leaves or flowers. Carefully dust off to rid the leaves of dirt and insects. Too much watering will remove the herb's essential oils. To dry herbs, hang them upside down in a cool, dry place with good airflow for 3 weeks before using.

Playing in the garden with these various methods will help you find diverse ways to make friends with the fae folk. Follow your intuition. Allow your instinct to guide you. Add to your wealth of innate knowledge by taking a glimpse at ancient herbal healing modalities.

Complementary Medicine

There are five main complementary healing modalities that use herbs: aroma therapy, Traditional Chinese Medicine, homeopathy, ayurveda, and herbalism. Although these healing modalities have different approaches, they all agree that the essence of plant medicine works on our emotional and physical bodies whether our mind-body is aware of what the plants are doing or not. Below is a summary of each of these holistic approaches to health and healing.

Aromatherapy is a practice first used by the ancient Chinese, Greeks, Romans, and Egyptians. It uses volatile liquid plant materials, known as essential oils, and other aromatic compounds from plants for cosmetics, massage, hygiene, medical treatments, and emotional needs. The volatile compounds can be extracted from flowers, leaves, roots, bark, seeds, and peels. Each of these essential oils is highly concentrated and has specific healing properties, including antibacterial, anti-inflammatory, antispasmodic, sedative, disinfectant, and antiviral. They can be soothing, antiseptic, antispasmodic, warming, or stimulating. Essential oils are used in several types of applications, including steam inhalation, dry inhalation, healing compresses, humidifiers, herbal saunas, or with a base or carrier oil for natural healing or beauty recipes.

Essential oils stimulate the nerves in the olfactory organs and are then transmitted to the parts of the brain that control emotions. Whether inhaled or absorbed through the skin, some oils are thought to reach the pituitary gland, which controls the adrenals that regulate stress and relaxation responses.

Carrier oils "carry" the potent essential oil for use on the skin. Carrier oils, such as almond, apricot kernel, olive, grapeseed, coconut, sesame, avocado, and jojoba oil, are fatty, plant-based oils. Most essential oils should be diluted with a carrier oil; the only exceptions are lavender and tea tree oil. Essential oils are hydrophobic, meaning they avoid water and prefer to cling to fat. Attempts to wash off essential oils should be done with a carrier oil; using soap and water will only cause the essential oil to absorb that much quicker into the fatty tissue of your skin.

Essential oils are available in a variety of places. Be an informed buyer and read labels when purchasing these oils. The quality of essential oils depends on the plant species, region, soil conditions, climate, time of day the plant material was harvested, and the method of extraction and storage. Organic, wildcrafted plant material is preferred, and steam distillation and cold-pressing are considered to be the best methods of extraction. In most cases, avoid perfumed, blended, reconstituted, or synthetic oils, or anything with chemical additives, particularly when your intention is to use the oils for healing. Again, it is the aliveness or life force of the plant that promotes health, not what is manufactured in chemical labs.

Traditional Chinese Medicine (TCM) has been practiced for thousands of years. TCM derives its theoretical and philosophical foundations from the book *The Yellow Emperor's Inner Classics*. This book was compiled between 200 BCE and 100 CE and remained the main source regarding the practice of herbal medicine for many years. (Modern titles include *The Yellow Emperor's Classic of Medicine: A*

New Translation, The Yellow Emperor's Canon of Medicine, and *The Yellow Emperor's Class of Internal Medicine.*)

The underlying philosophy of this ancient text was the view that disease was the manifestation of malevolent spirits, ghosts, or demons, which must be repelled by incarnation, rituals, and spells in addition to herbal prescriptions. Medicines had to be empowered by words, rituals, and sacred space and time. The aromatic smells of such herbs as cinnamon bark and mugwort were considered to have magical properties that affected demons or a person's own spiritual powers. As time went on, people began to better understand the natural world and that health and disease were subject to the principles of the natural order instead of the mercy of spirits, ghosts, and demons.

Modern TCM practitioners view people and the universe as composed of various forces based on the complementary opposites of *yin* and *yang* and the five elements: wood, water, fire, earth, and metal. Health and illness are considered a natural phenomenon, and natural law operates upon the cosmos, humans, and the connection between them.

To promote the flow of *qi*, TCM practitioners use a variety of methods such as acupuncture, acupressure, Tuina massage, qi gong (breathing in sync with specific exercises), tai chi, nutritional and lifestyle counseling, and herbal medicine.

The most common way of using herbs for healing is a tea decoction. Often herbs are added to soup broth, and then rice, meat, and veggies are added when the herbs are cooked and removed. The herbs are boiled for a specific amount of time and a certain number of times, and either added together or taken separately, depending on the disease or imbalance. TCM also uses tinctures, powders, honey pills, capsules, and tablets to administer herbal formulas internally. Externally, the herbs are delivered in the form of plasters, oils, compresses both hot and cold, salves, lotions, oils in the ear, gargles, steams, and moxibustion (burning herbs on or near the skin); this last practice must be performed by a qualified practitioner only.

TCM practitioners observe the reactions to, as well as the taste, temperature, toxicity, function, primary clinical applications, processing, and preparation of, herbal medicine. Information regarding reactions is gathered from a patient's description of how he or she feels and from clinical observations of a patient after ingesting an herb or combination of herbs. Tastes are based on five flavors: savory, sweet, bitter, sour, and salty. According to TCM, savoriness travels in the qi and enters the lungs; sweetness travels in the flesh and enters the spleen; bitterness travels in the bones and enters the heart; sourness travels in the sinews and enters the liver; and saltiness travels in the blood and enters the kidneys. Temperature is determined by how an herb either feels on the skin or how it makes the body react after ingesting the herb. There are hot, warm, cool, cold, and neutral herbs. Each disease or condition is treated with its "opposite" herb: a hot disease is treated with cold herbs. A cold disease is treated with hot herbs. A warm disease is treated with cool herbs, and a cool disease is treated with warm herbs. The function of an herb is based on the nature of the herb's energy to rise, fall, float, or sink. Also, an herb's function is based on the organ that the herb has an affinity for, whether it goes to the lung, large intestine, stomach, spleen, heart, small intestine, urinary bladder, kidney, pericardium, triple burner, gallbladder, or liver. Another way of determining the function of an herb in Chinese herbal medicine is by its use in the eight therapeutic methods: promoting sweating, inducing vomiting, purging, harmonizing, warming, clearing, tonifying, and reducing. The action of the herb also determines how an herb is used—i.e., whether it is an herb that is dissipating, unblocking, tonifying, purging, slippery and lubricating, astringent, drying, moistening, light, heavy, hot, cold, ascending, or descending.

TCM is based on a holistic approach to health, and so the patient is observed and interviewed to see where the imbalance is located and the type of disease: exterior or interior, hot or cold, due to excess or deficiency, and finally whether it is yin or yang. Which organ or channels the imbalance affects also plays into the equation. Herbal combinations are created for their mutual accentuation, mutual enhancement, mutual counteraction, mutual suppression, mutual antagonism, mutual incompatibility, and single effect. Cautions and contraindications must be heeded as well as combination prohibitions and dietary incompatibilities. All these factors have to be determined before a formula can be developed for the patient.

Homeopathy treats disease and/or discomfort with heavily diluted preparations that are thought to cause effects similar to the disease's symptoms. First expounded by German physician Samuel Hahnemann in 1796, homeopathic remedies (also called homeopathics) are a system of medicine based on nine principles: like cures like, minimal doses, single remedy, vital force, susceptibility, miasms, provings, potentizations, and totality. To stimulate the body's natural ability to heal itself, homeopathic practitioners administer tiny amounts of substances that would otherwise produce similar symptoms to the ailment. The remedy is taken in an extremely diluted form. No matter how many symptoms are experienced, only one remedy is taken, and that remedy will be aimed at all those symptoms. Vital force refers to the life energy that animates every living being. Susceptibility is a person's resistance to disease. Miasms are a person's inherited predisposition to develop certain types of disease. Provings refer to the tests of remedies to establish their effectiveness. Potentization is the unique process by which homoeopathic remedies are made with repeated dilution and shaking. Totality means considering the entire picture of a person's symptoms and physical, mental, and emotional states.

Homeopathic remedies are made from plants, animals, and minerals. They are most often made into tablets, usually in a base of lactose or sucrose, and taken under the tongue, where the medicine can be quickly absorbed into the bloodstream. More than 3,000 known remedies are available to encourage the body's natural defense system and promote health and healing.

The underlying principle of "like cures like" is similar to the basis of conventional allergy treatment, where the allergic substance is given in a small dose, and in vaccines, where an impotent form of the virus is given to bolster the immune system against that particular virus. This is yet another example of allowing the life force to develop in strength and, through vitality, create health and healing.

Homeopathy is the second most widely used system of medicine in the world. Its growth in popularity in the United States has been around 25 to 50 percent a year throughout the past decade. This success is fueled by its effectiveness and safety (even babies and pregnant women can use homeopathy without the danger of side effects). Homeopathy is natural and works in harmony with your immune system.

Ayurveda originated in India during the Vedic period, the second and first millennia BCE. It is said that the Hindu god Brahma revealed the system of Ayurveda, or "the knowledge of long life." In Sanskrit, the word *Ayurveda* comprises the words *yus*, meaning "life" and *veda*, meaning "science." At the heart of Ayurveda is the belief that those who live in harmony with nature and the totality of their being are healthy. According to Ayurvedic principles, people and nature are linked by the five elements: fire, water, air, earth, and ether, which are expressed in the three life forces known as *doshas: vata, pitta,* and *kapha.*

To harmonize a person's dosha, Ayurvedic practitioners apply massage and affusions or recommend diet or life changes and herbal remedies. The three doshas are defined as follows: vata personalities are wiry, small-boned, nervous, and usually quickly roused; pitta types are medium-boned, strong, determined, and quick-tempered; and kapha types are athletic, stocky, slow-moving, and generally emotionally stable. Ayurveda uses herbs and plants to eliminate the excess or waste in the body and weaken the deficiencies with the principles of the five elements. Ayurveda considers the broader energetic effects of the herbs on overall metabolic processes.

The properties of herbs are related systematically according to their taste, elements, heating or cooling effects, effects after digestion, and other special potencies.

Ayurvedic practitioners consider sickness a result of an imbalance among the doshas. They begin with a comprehensive interview and examination that takes into consideration the person's body structure, nutrition, lifestyle, spirituality, Ayurvedic pulse diagnosis, and palpation of important parts of the body, such as the fingernails, tongue, and eyes.

A particularly common and effective practice in Ayurveda is *panchakarma*, which uses a broad set of five cleansing therapies and is a personalized three-, five-, or 7-day detoxification and rejuvenation process, according to the individual's imbalanced state of mind and body, to eliminate the accumulated toxins. The process starts with a very broad inquiry into a person's health and lifestyle history to understand how he or she is prone, or vulnerable, to various maladies. Based on this understanding, an overall therapy plan is prepared, including pre-therapy supplements, exercises, diet, etc., followed by hands-on therapy administration, followed by an at-home, self-therapy plan.

Panchakarma is a holistic, health-giving series of therapeutic treatments that cleanse the body's deep tissues of toxins; open the subtle channels; bring life-enhancing energy; eliminate toxins and toxic conditions from your body and mind; restore your constitutional balance, improving health and wellness; strengthen your immune system; reverse the negative effects of stress on your body and mind; promote longevity, self-reliance, strength, energy, vitality, and mental clarity; and induce deep relaxation and a sense of well-being. Panchakarma is an ongoing process that continues even after the initial treatment.

Herbalism is an ancient method of healing based on the use of herbs, trees, and plant or tree extracts. Herbalism is also known as herbology, botanical medicine, medical herbalism, or herbal medicine. The scope of herbal medicine can also include fungal and bee products, as well as minerals, shells, and certain animal parts.

Herbalists traditionally use fresh herbs in their healing practice. Their forms of treatment include infusions, teas, decoctions, tinctures, poultices, washes, ointments, and herbal-infused oils. Many herbalists grow their own herbs and have long, well-developed relationships with the plants. The preference to work directly with the plants, rather than with essential oils or some other form, is based on the fact that whole herbs have more of the life force pulsating through them. Over years of gardening and creating their own concoctions, herbalists constantly discover new ways to apply their herbs and how the seasons or weather affects their plants and patients.

With each turn of the Wheel of the Year, all herbal healing practitioners become a little closer to the fae energy of the herbs they work with—they learn a little more about the faerie's message.

Although there are several ways to work with herbs that will satisfy medical, emotional, or spiritual issues, teas are the most common and easily accessible form to use. An herbal tea is typically 1 tablespoon of herb to 1 cup (250 milliliters) of water. To increase its potency, a weak infusion can be made with ½ ounce of herb in 1 pint (500 milliliters) of water for 15 minutes. A medium-strength infusion consists of steeping ⅔ ounce of herb in 1 pint (500 milliliters) of water for an hour. For a strong medical infusion, steep 1 ounce of herb in 1 pint (500 milliliters) of water overnight. Drain the herbs by placing a cloth inside a colander, preserving the strained water. Once most of the water has drained through, squeeze the cloth.

The Faeries' Message

Everlasting Life

As we connect on a deeper level with the faeries, we will gain access to the wisdom of these spirits. As spirits of the earth, faeries live as the earth lives. In other words, they are immortal. The elemental realm exists in a parallel universe to our own, interacting beside our own. Just as the indigenous animals and birds live next to you as you go to work, take a walk through a park, or go to the grocery store, the elemental world is experiencing life right next to you.

The fae folk are cavorting, squeezing the juice out of life, enticing you to play—at all times. They hide things to bring them back miraculously—particularly keys. Have you ever noticed? They ensure our favorite flowers bloom just when we need an emotional boost. They make the wind chimes tinkle to let us know we're not alone. They try to get us to have some fun, but many of us have distanced ourselves from the concept of play, relying instead on serious work as the best way to establish security and safety. The truth is, we wouldn't be so concerned about our security if we trusted our foundation more—the earth and the elemental beings who are waiting to be our teachers. The faeries are eager to develop a bond they once knew with their human brothers and sisters. If we accepted the mystery and magick that surround us, we'd take a collective sigh of relief and begin to trust again.

Reintroduce yourself to the very spirits of Mother Earth: the plant devas, the faeries, and the dryads who are here to teach us play, heal, and love. They want us to remember that as children of the universe we are not only allowed to play but are also encouraged to be playful and silly. In fact, the root of the word *silly* comes from the Germanic word *selig*, meaning "holy." The art of playing with the earth is a sacred act. Whereas crying cleanses our emotional body, playfulness and laughter cleanse our soul. It is our divine right to be playful. The fae do not have the rules that we have. To experience magick, look to the heavens and gaze upon the stars that blanket the sky. Notice how the open laughter of a small child or gentle hug of a soft breeze gives life fuel for one more day.

The faeries have watched us, and through their compassion for us, they have yearned for us to understand that we are like them—children of nature. They want us to know that as their brothers and sisters, we are related, and so we are also eternal beings.

For a moment, consider this: you are an eternal being.

When you recognize yourself as an everlasting soul, if you know that deep in your core you and your loved ones will never die, then, truly, there is nothing to fear. As an eternal being, you will have opportunities to experience everything, from climbing the tallest mountains to being male or female, victim or victor. With an understanding that you live on an endless continuum, you will not need to rush any moment. Each outcome will naturally flow to you. The idea of living in the moment, appreciating the presence, will come so much easier when you place less value on time.

Before someone taught you to read a clock, time was measured in moments that could be quick, like a chase through the meadows, or very slow, like ambling down a lazy river on a raft. Days varied in their length according to the experiences we had. We lived each moment for the bliss it gave us and never worried about when the next moment would come or how long this one would last, or what we should do to make sure it stayed securely locked in our memories. We just played. Close your eyes and take a moment to remember a time without worries. Slowly, a smile will bless your face and with it a feeling of wellness bubbling from deep within your soul.

What if we listened to every elder who said that life goes by too fast and decided right then and there not to waste another moment on worry or fear? You'd let every hurt go and focus primarily on the joy waiting to burst forth. You'd focus more on what is going right in your life, rather than give your attention to the reasons for complaint. And in this way, you can be assured of health in your everlasting life.

Feel Good to Attract More of the Same

Science has proven that we are more energy than matter. We are more spirit than physical. And yet, we often get stuck trying to force life into preconceived notions of the proper ways things can show up. Faerie energy reminds us to concentrate on the essence, the juicy, vibrant feelings of life. Happiness is not found in things but in attitude. Faeries are ephemeral beings that want us to remember the feeling of biting into a mango or walking barefoot through mud after a refreshing spring rain. These experiences bring us back to a time when the dividing line between us and nature was nothing real, nothing tangible. We are one with the earth.

What would life feel like if we were able to dance without risk of judgment or being ostracized? What if you could give in to the visions and instincts that allow us to communicate with all spirit life that lives upon this earth?

Any and every experience or feeling is yours for the having as long as you allow your attention to settle on it. When you feel the strength of the good feelings, you will attract more of the same to you. And imagine if society held no concept of shame, pity, or duty. In the elemental world, the fae folk have no need for these life-draining feelings. As the earth's spirit, fae energy naturally goes toward the exquisite, the height of ecstasy, the best that life has to offer. What if you were free, empowered to choose your experiences without fear of condemnation? What if you could aspire for your most brazen wish without worrying about someone else feeling small or abandoned or jealous? Our natural inclination, our knee-jerk reaction as children, was to see ourselves and life through rose-colored glasses. We splashed in water puddles, rolled down grassy hills, and laughed until our bellies ached. We knew we were the creators of our reality, and we naturally chose good feelings. Before someone explained right or wrong, we chose what felt good and though we had no moral compass, we rarely went beyond impish.

Faeries know that the overall good of the human and faerie tribes relies upon our ability to flow with life—to play with the elements and follow the prana or breath with ease. Any faerie will tell you that there is no need for struggle. Faeries do not fight nature. They do not dam rivers or plant trees that do not feed indigenous creatures. They work with nature—aligning their desires, their play, into the natural order of the cosmos.

And when a desire sparks within the wee faeries' mind, they employ the art of wishing, which begins with a focused intention, dropping into the feeling they want to manifest and a knowing that they have every right to happiness—in fact, they never even consider whether or not they deserve it. They believe that life is supposed to be infused with the beauty and richness of nature's perfect balance and are accustomed to that effortless well-being. They trust that if something feels good, then of course it will come around again. Their expectation makes it so.

The natural world is verdant and abundant. Trees, bushes, herbs, soil, stone, rivers, lakes, and the seas teem with a strong life force. This vitality is self-renewing and points out the abundance that is available for the taking. There is so much to choose from, so much lush experience to dive into. Faeries' willingness to trust in their inherent right to pleasure always attracts the feeling to them.

Faeries are drawn by the essence, feeling, or spirit of their desire. We often attach to a precise image of what our manifested wish will look like—whether we yearn for more love, better health, or greater prosperity. If we are to find true happiness and perfect physical and mental well-being, we must release the idea of how something needs to show up or how it looks and instead concentrate on how we will feel once our desires have been met.

Accept the Fluidity and Transitory Nature of Time

The world of faerie exists in twilight, time-space reality. Faeries comprise an elemental society, the essence of nature, an energy that is fleeting, transitory as shadow. What we thought was there moves and changes shape constantly, consistently. Faeries wink out by setting their focus on another place, and in a flash, they're gone. Their quick decisions change as the wind moves. As the essence of nature, faeries are the reflection of the natural world and so represent life's continual mode of change.

Faeries do not attach to form. They wish for a chair and it appears just for the time required—no more, no less. For us humans, we create things from thought and desire as well. The difference is, the things we create often outlast the desire. And when the time comes that we outgrow what we have created, we have difficulty letting go. We must learn from the fae who accept and enjoy the release.

Just look out your window and you'll see the wisdom of the faerie message to accept the fluidity and transitory nature of time. Observe the moon in its changing phases: an iridescent crescent, growing into glowing, ripe fullness, then receding into dark with a shimmering outline. The wind can blow chill or warm, soft or dangerous. The tide comes in, then ebbs out again, shifting the sand, changing the look of the beach with each movement of water and silt.

Faerie energy teaches us to accept this change inherent in nature and in life. It is pointless and exhausting to fight against change. It is much more prudent, relaxing, and empowering to simply close your eyes and ride the wind, travel atop the waves of life, and flow with and through the seasons of life. This constant movement is not a personal attack, a cruel joke of the Universe to throw you off center; rather, this call to movement is what keeps you from being static, becoming poisonous, like brackish,

THE FAERIES SPEAK

"Welcome to our world. We have waited for you, knowing our connection would bring you back again. We offer our gifts with love; by trusting us to be your guides you honor us with your attention. As the changes on Mother Earth continue, we rejoice in your awareness of her needs as well as your own. Through your journey in this book we would like to introduce you to not only our physical qualities but our magickal selves as well. Like most things, there is more to us than meets the eye. We have a connection that goes beyond the leaves and oils, beyond the branches and spices. Our time has finally come to be revealed.

Thank you for hearing us.

Now let us be introduced!"

still waters. We are children of nature and each day our body recreates itself. We must move with the changes or get run over in the process. Holding on to a moment will always make us miss what is around the next corner, which, believe it or not, could be better than the last.

Faeries implore us to trust the natural perpetual movement. To be free spirits, to let go of preconceptions, and to release judgment is what the faeries desire for us. Only with this lighthearted confidence and faith can life become a dance, a weaving around the maypole—enjoying a partner for as long as the moment lasts—never pining for an individual or a certain picture of how life should be. Faeries know that a fixed idea limits our ability to tap into the illimitable source that connects us all. Faeries have no need for ownership because they recognize themselves in everything. There are no dividing lines, no boundaries that separate us from nature. Faeries recognize what we must acknowledge: we are not merely part of nature; we are nature. To feel this connection is to know joy. When you feel joy, only health and healing can be in your mind, body, and soul.

To begin this journey, let's meet thirty-three favorite herbs and trees of the garden. Get to know them. Plant them. Eat them. Speak to them. Dance with them. Love them.

Herb Index

The relationship between human and plant was considered so sacred by ancient healers that it was recommended that apprentices work with only one plant at a time. Only when the link between human and plant had become so tight and secure could the student move on to another plant. This process could take months; it could take years. For this reason, we have included a small number of herbs to help you get acquainted with their healing, magickal, and medicinal properties, growing conditions, and faerie essences.

We hope to break down any trepidation you may have in working with herbs by helping you recognize friends in the plant world. With a connection to a particular faerie, you might find a comrade in naughty deeds or a teacher in compassion. You will find which plants bring calm, which ones revitalize, which ones are good for the skin, and which herbs add spice to your life. Each body has its own complex configuration, so you will find in nature that several herbs alleviate the same ailment. There are far few panaceas in this world. You must try the different herbs and discover which brings you comfort—lavender or chamomile—and which brings relief to your cough—mullein or eucalyptus. With a deep connection to your plant kindom and your own intuition, you will find the right combination for you. The faeries invite you to trust yourself.

Thirty-three herbs were chosen to get you started on your journey into green magick in the garden. Thirty-three is a profoundly magickal number and was chosen for its inherent mystic and powerful symbolism. It is considered a master number. Both Alexander the Great and Jesus Christ died at the age of thirty-three. Three is the number that represents manifestation and creation, simply by virtue of the fact that it takes one female and one male to create one child. Thirty-three doubles that numeral and thereby increases your ability to create magick. It also corresponds to the number of points in the ancient symbol of the overlapping apex and vortex triangles, also known as the Star of David. The apex triangle points to the sky and is typically considered yang, male, or active energy, whereas the vortex triangle points to the earth and is generally yin, female, or resting energy. The intersection is where magick happens.

These particular herbs were chosen because of their common use in culinary recipes, natural beauty supplies, and medicinal remedies. They can be found in your garden or neighborhood. They are readily available at most garden nurseries or in the spice section of the grocery store. Over the past several years we have developed a sacred relationship with each of these herbs, having grown them in the garden, used them as ingredients for lotions and potions, called upon their medicine to heal us or our loved ones, and cooked fabulous dishes with them.

There will be an image of each of the faerie essences accompanied by the faerie's message. Practical information includes common name, Latin name, folk names, parts used, description, growing conditions, faerie essence, lore, associations, traditional uses, ritual, home remedy, or meditation, as well as a culinary, natural beauty, medicinal, or magickal recipe. A combination of mysticism and practical information will help herbal enthusiasts from all levels better relate to these common plants and trees, the individual faerie or life force, and the gifts they offer.

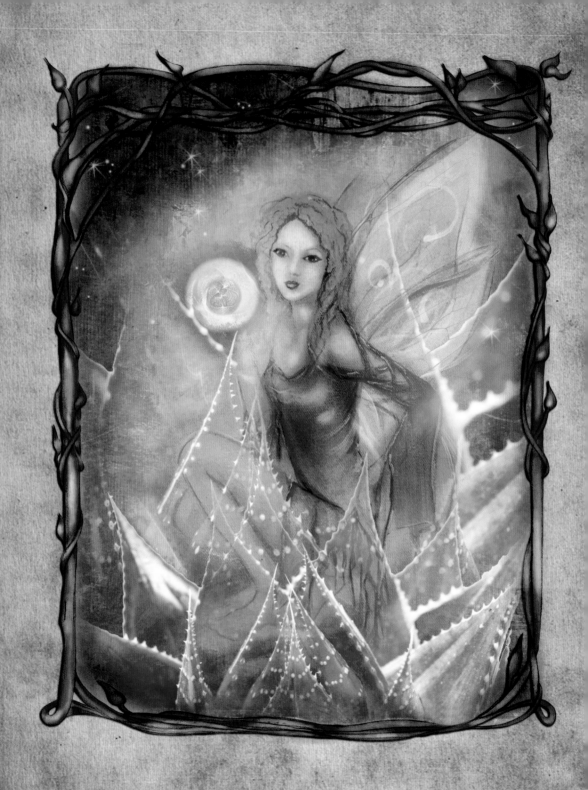

Aloe

Aloe vera

Aloes, Aloe Vera, Burn Plant, Medicine Plant

PARTS USED: LEAVES

Aloe leaves are sage green and grow wand-like, with spines along the sides to protect the plant from grazing animals. Red-orange flowers tipped with yellow shoot up in warmer months. Aloe is usually found in dry, sandy, and rocky regions. It likes full sun or light shade inland. Water deeply, but infrequently. Grow in loose, dry, well-drained soil rich in humus in reasonably frost-free areas.

Aloe is one of the easiest and most successful plants to propagate. When the leaves of the offshoot begin to unfold and form a rosette, they are suitable for propagation. Remove the potting mix around the offshoot and follow it back to the base of the aloe. Pull it up gently and look for any roots that may already be coming from the offshoot. Use caution to keep these roots intact because they do give the propagation a head start. However, aloe will still replant well without a root system. Plant in a 3-inch pot with standard potting mix, then add a $1/2$-inch layer of sand on top of the potting mix.

ALOE

"I am the first to meet, my pleasure to greet. Don't let my rough exterior fool you. I am gentle inside: It is where I hide all of my delicate juices that soothe you."

Aloe is best known for its ability to relieve the pain of burns. It is believed to bring love and companionship to the lonely. In fact, due to its ability to survive in harsh conditions and yet sustain a soothing quality, the faerie essence of aloe is success and harmony. To further enhance this particular feeling, aloe resonates with both Venus and Mars, balancing the energy of male/action and female/rest. This plant brings synergy to complicated or discordant relationships and situations. It assists the transformation of pain and suffering into vitality and well-being. Sheathed in spines, the healing power of aloe's calming coolness is well guarded, thus giving it protection as an herb and an energy.

Do not use aloe internally if you are pregnant.

Aloe is also used to treat gastrointestinal ailments, as a diuretic and blood cleanser, and to boost the immune system. Aloe can be taken as a laxative in small doses. Aloe juice taken one tablespoon a day prior to your menses will help alleviate blood clots.

Soothing Lip Balm

Aloe enjoys a long history of medicinal use and is considered to be the only plant to come directly from the Garden of Eden. Traditionally, it was hung over the doorway of travelers to ensure safety on their journeys. The plant is strongly associated with the prophet Mohammed. It has been used as a funeral herb for centuries, and is even believed to have been used in the wrappings of Christ's body. Interestingly, aloe is planted on graves to bring peace to the deceased until their resurrection. It is also buried with the placentas of babies to reinforce their connection with the earth. The extra nutrients of the placenta that feed the soil will go into the aloe and extend its healing properties. Because aloe has been used to soothe, protect, and heal, its innate soothing qualities will enhance the lip balm recipe provided below.

INGREDIENTS

3 tablespoons beeswax
3 tablespoons aloe vera gel
2 tablespoons coconut oil
8 drops lavender essential oil

Bring the water to a boil in the bottom of a double boiler. Place the beeswax in a jar and place in the top portion of the double boiler. Once the beeswax has melted, combine the remaining ingredients in a small glass bowl. Mix well, and pour into a 4-ounce (113-milliliter) container. Let cool completely. Store in a dark place.

Yields ¹/₂ cup (113 milliliters)

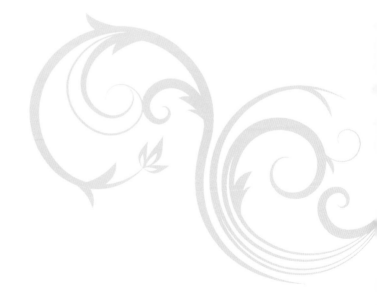

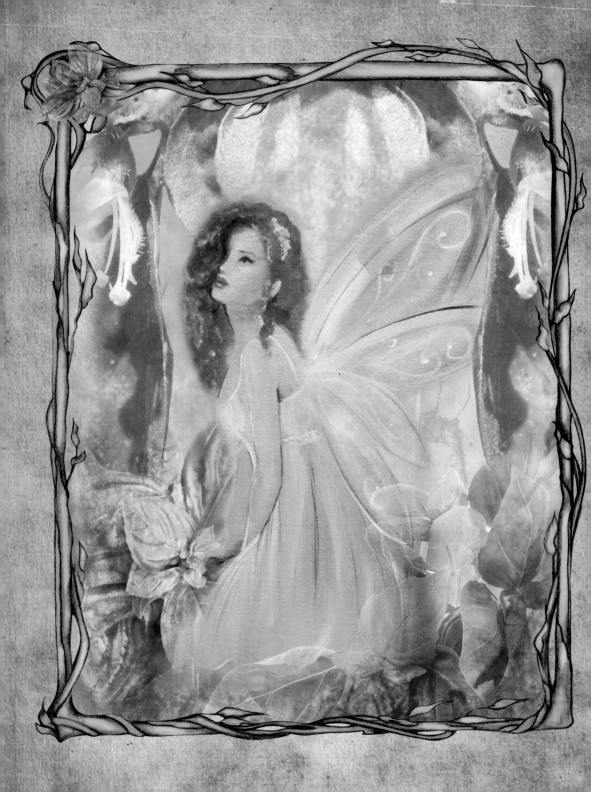

Basil

Ocimum basilicum

Alabahaca, American Dittany, Our Herb, St. Joseph's Wort, Witches' Herb

PARTS USED: LEAVES, FLOWERS

Basil has whorls of small, white-hooded flowers and shiny, bright green oval leaves. It is found in woodlands and in many gardens. This annual herb prefers full sun and regular watering; occasional, overhead watering will produce bright, clean foliage. Sow basil seed in early spring, planting successively 2 weeks apart. Space the plants 10 to 12 inches apart. Fertilize once during the summer months with a balanced fertilizer.

Drinking basil tea can relieve nausea, vomiting, and indigestion and stimulate the immune system. The leaves can be rubbed on the skin to relieve bites from snakes, scorpions, and spiders. You can add basil, along with oregano and a bay leaf, to olive oil for your own special culinary oil. Due to its warming quality, in Ayurvedic medicine basil is used to relieve chills, coughs, snakebites, skin irritations and infections, and earaches. The fae energy of this plant is a quiet, warming strength.

Do not use basil oil extensively with toddlers or pregnant women.

Basil is associated with Brigid's Day, a fire holiday celebrated on February 1 or 2. Brigid is an ancient Celtic goddess known for ruling over smith crafting, poetry, and fire. She is also associated with inspiration, wells, health, healing, new endeavors, and opportunities. On her holiday, candles are burned and flowers are brought to sacred wells all over Ireland. The wells are symbolic of the cauldron, chalice, or womb—the birthplace of creation. Followers of Brigid have tended her sacred fire for hundreds of years. It is no wonder that her holy day of fire falls on the first day of February, a time of year when the sun is gaining in strength, yet winter still clings to the land and the need for fire is so strong.

BASIL

"Hello! The sun is out and just as I play upon your tongue, it beckons us to dance. Dance with me, then, and savor my company, as I do yours."

A protector who can purify any space, Brigid was so beloved by the Celtic pagans when the Christians took over, around 500 CE they could not erase Brigid from the hearts of the people, and so they absorbed her almost literally into the Christian faith as St. Brigid. Her holiday morphed into Candlemas (candle mass), sometimes known as Imbolc ("in milk," which is a reference to the fact that animals such as sheep were giving birth and lactating), and eventually known in America as Groundhog's Day, a day simply for divination of weather—will the light of the sun cast a shadow, foretelling how long winter will last?

Basil's fae essence combines the protection, creativity, and inspiration of Brigid with the herb's other qualities. Use basil to promote peace, protection, purification, cleansing, tranquility, business success, love, and money. It is also used to uplift the spirits and has antidepressant qualities.

Baked Salmon with Citrus Pesto Sauce

INGREDIENTS

I bunch fresh basil
¹/₂ cup (113 grams) pine nuts
I clove garlic
I lemon, zested and juiced
I orange, zested and juiced
¹/₂ teaspoon salt
¹/₂ teaspoon pepper

¹/₂ cup (125 milliliters) canola oil
I cup (228 grams) grated
    parmesan cheese
I salmon fillet
Salt and freshly ground pepper
I lemon
I lime

Blend the basil, pine nuts, garlic, zests, juices, salt, and pepper in a food processor until the mixture is finely chopped. Add the canola oil and continue to blend until the mixture is smooth and creamy. Transfer to a bowl and stir in the parmesan. Refrigerate the citrus pesto sauce, covered, until ready to serve.

Cover a baking sheet with foil. Place the salmon on the baking sheet and season generously with salt and pepper. Cut the lemon and lime in half. Use half of each for juice, squeezing over the salmon. Slice the remaining halves into thin slivers and cover the salmon. Bake at 350°F (177°C) for 25 minutes. Serve with the citrus pesto spooned on top.

Serves 2

Note: Before you begin, sit for a moment in stillness. Be aware of your body and breathe gently but deeply. Whenever you cook, whether it is a lotion, potion, or fantastic meal, your intention is an essential ingredient. Your energy literally pours into the bowl and mixes in with everything else.

This recipe was donated by aspiring chef Brian Regan.

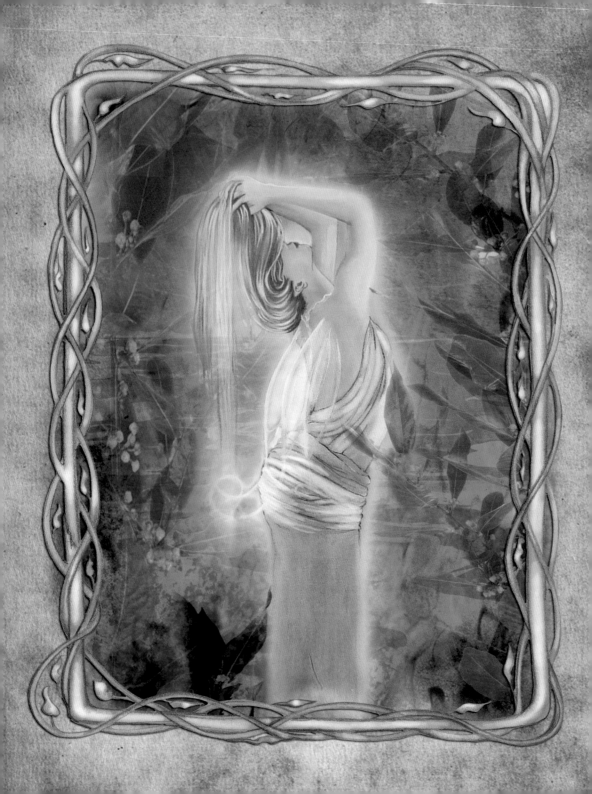

Bay Laurel

Laurus nobilis

Bay, Bay Tree, Daphne, Grecian Laurel, Roman Laurel, Sweet Bay

PARTS USED: LEAVES

Bay leaves are oval, shiny, and gold flecked. The flowers are round and green, and the berries are dark. Bay trees prefer Mediterranean climates that provide moderate temperature, soil that drains well, and ample sunlight. They are somewhat difficult to root, so it is advisable to begin with a young tree from a reputable nursery.

Bay laurel is associated with the Greek god Apollo, who is in charge of pulling the sun across the sky. The ancient Greeks rewarded their victorious athletes with a crown of bay leaves and stories that would regale their victories for millennia to come. Bay was once used by the priestesses of Delphi as a visionary herb to help them with prophecy, but under extreme care, because this is quite a dangerous practice. It was also used in rituals of love and self-esteem. Thus, it has become tradition to associate bay faerie energy with victory, meditation, love, clairvoyance, success, and prosperity. Today, some people put three bay leaves into wish boxes to give their desire an extra push toward manifestation.

Bay leaves are a natural remedy for the painful itching of stinging nettle and poison oak or poison ivy. It is wondrous to note that the remedy often grows next to the poison. For a quick cure, you can add a fistful of bay leaves to a kettle of boiling water and allow them to steep for 10 minutes. Apply with a cotton ball or washcloth, or if you have neither of those just pour warm tea over the infected area. If the affected area is small, simply crush three or four leaves and rub the leaves over the skin. The volatile oils will take the sting out. Bay leaves can also be added to a bowl of steaming water to energize tired feet.

Due to bay's history of being associated with victory and success, it has been used as a powerful herb in many prosperity and money rituals. As you create this recipe, think about the success you want to bring to your life and all the good money can do for you.

Money likes to be circulated—that's why coins are round. Money was not intended to be hoarded but to be in constant motion. For above all, money is energy. Like water, stagnate energy turns poisonous, but with constant movement, it can produce amazing and beautiful results. If you pay attention, you'll notice that money literally falls from the sky. With just a little awareness, you could find a coin on the ground every day. Pick it up. Do your part to keep money in circulation, because money is to be shared to bring about more wealth, more success.

When you imagine money coming to you, think also about how the money you receive will positively affect other people. For example, let's say you need $500 to fix your car. With a running car, you could give a friend a ride to school. And with the extra time the friend saves by not having to walk, she could spend more time volunteering at the hospital where she visits the elderly. And then the elderly would feel loved and perhaps energized by the attention and find a bit more health. They would be kinder and gentler to everyone around them, who would in turn be kinder and gentler to the next person. See how far you can extrapolate and imagine what good that mere $500 can bring to the world.

Prosperity Soup

As you make this recipe for your family or a group of friends, repeat this phrase either during the process of making the soup or while serving, or both:

"Prosperity is our divine right.
Bless us, Apollo, with your Light.
Security and Abundance are in Sight."

INGREDIENTS

¹/₂ cup (113 grams) chopped yellow onion
2 cloves garlic, minced
2 tablespoons butter
2 cups (500 grams) white beans
2 quarts (2 liters) water
2 bay leaves
2 teaspoons chopped basil
1 tablespoon honey
Salt and freshly ground pepper
1 tablespoon olive oil
¹/₂ cup (113 grams) chopped parsley
2 green onions, chopped

BAY LAUREL

"If you would let me, I would wrap myself around your head, and crown you champion of this day. If it pleases you I will soothe your aching feet, remove the sting from neighboring plants, and shower you with the energy of abundance. Your wish is my destiny."

Sauté the onion and garlic in butter until soft, stirring often. Add the beans, water, bay leaves, basil, and honey. Bring the mixture to a boil, reduce to a simmmer, and cover. Continue cooking until the beans are tender, about 2 hours, adding more water if necessary, and stirring occasionally. Season with salt and pepper. While the soup is cooling, purée the beans in a blender or food processor. Return the puréed soup to the pot, and reheat over moderate heat, stirring often. Blend in the olive oil. Garnish with parsley and green onions, and serve hot.

Serves 4

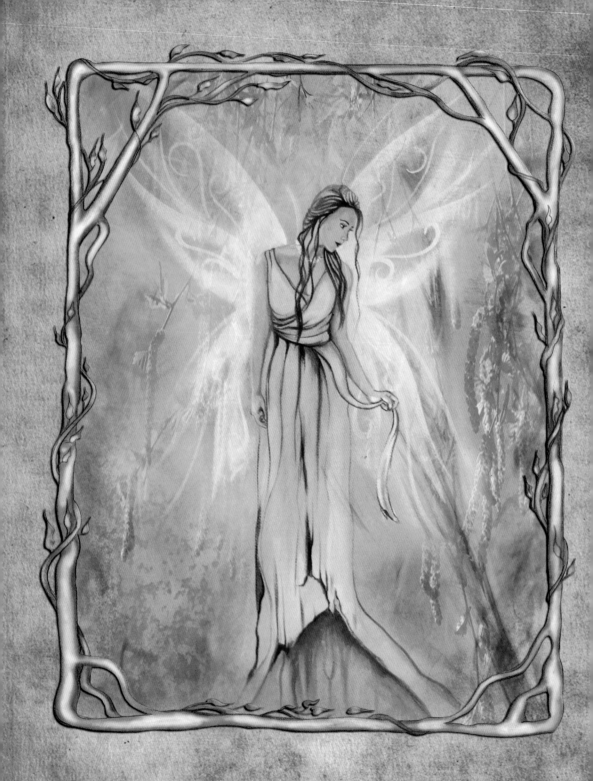

Birch

Betula (various species)

Lady of the Woods, Mountain Mahogany

PARTS USED: LEAVES, BUDS, CATKINS, BARK, BRANCHES

The birch is a deciduous tree with small, fine-toothed, serrated leaves. The bark of all birches is characteristically marked with long horizontal lenticels, and often separates into thin papery plates. Birch trees prefer full sun and rainy climates or ample watering.

Birch embodies the fae essence of awakening, "tabula rasa," a blank slate or fresh start in accordance with its traditional use as paper and its connection to certain deities. Where the tree grew, birch bark was among the first paper traditional people used. Birch itself became a symbol, Beth or the letter B, for the early alphabet of the British Isles. The birch tree has been important to many cultures throughout history. It is associated with Thor, the Norse God of War, who used his hammer Mjolnir to break up the ice of winter each spring. Also associated with Venus, the Roman Goddess of Spring, birch symbolizes the bridge between the darkness of winter and the rebirth and stirrings of spring. Birch represents the importance of your awareness during the moment of awakening. As you transition from unknowing to the fullness of your fresh new self, your focused attention allows for the fullness of experience to live in you on a deep, visceral level.

Birch can be applied to open wounds and skin irritations. It is an effective diuretic, antiseptic, tonic, and detergent. The oil, which dissipates quickly when exposed to heat, can be used as an aftershave, lotion, or massage oil. Beer can be made from the inner bark of the sweet birch (*Betula lenta*). Native Americans made syrup from the sap of the tree. Fallen birch branches are a frequent choice for wand making. Because birch is connected to beginnings, its trunk has traditionally been used as maypoles for Beltane celebrations. It is highly regarded as a protective tree, and thus its branches have been constructed into baby cradles for centuries.

Sometimes known as Lady of the Woods, birch aids in communicating with the energy of the woods and forests, particularly the faun known as Pan, the Greek God of Nature. Meditating in a grove of birch trees will bring inspiration and clarity to muddled or confusing situations.

Birch Blessings Incantation

Anoint a piece of parchment paper with birch oil and write down an intention or wish. Roll the paper toward you in a symbolic gesture of calling your desire to you. Combine 2 ounces (60 grams) of a carrier oil (such as jojoba, almond, apricot, or extra virgin olive oil) with 4 drops birch oil. Rub the oil on your hands and say:

"I draw to me the wish of my heart.
Knowing myself as whole, not part."

Hold your hands to the sky, like you're catching falling leaves of happiness from the birch tree, and say:

"Of Earth and her treasures within,
I call this moment to begin."

Draw the energy down from the tips of the topmost leaf, down through the caress of a silvery trunk. Imagine your fingers filling with dirt as you reach for her roots. Rub the oil on your feet. Repeat three times:

"I walk the path of my dreams.
I draw positive energy into me.
This I make true, three times three times three."

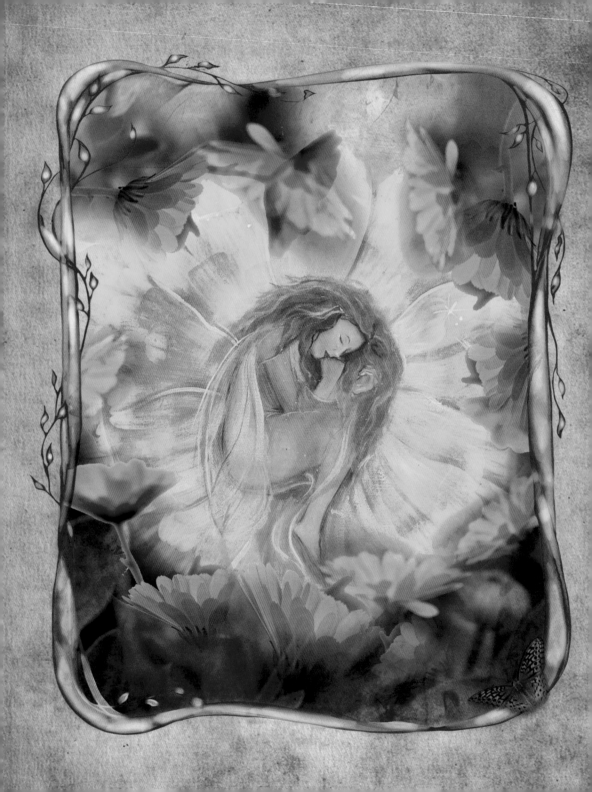

Calendula

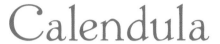

Calendula officinalis

Bride of the Sun, Gold Bloom, Pot Marigold, Summer's Bride

PARTS USED: FLOWERS, LEAVES

Calendula is recognized for its bright yellow flowers, resembling the sun. The leaves are pale green and oval. It flourishes in warm, sunny locations, although it can also thrive in shade. It grows well in any soil, even heavy clay. It is best to plant in fall or early spring. The flowers are edible and have a peppery taste.

It is important to be certain you do not confuse calendula with the plant typically called marigold, which has the Latin name *Tagetes*; for the most part, the *Tagetes* species are toxic.

Although it is best known for its skin-soothing properties and its exceptional power to heal wounds due to its cleansing, astringent, and antifungal effects, calendula has also been used to induce prophetic dreams. It was once believed that if you rubbed a concoction of calendula and honey over your body before going to sleep, your future mate would appear in a dream.

The word *calendula* originates from the Latin word *calends*, the first day of the Roman month. The nickname pot marigold comes from the Virgin Mary combined with the precious metal gold. Due to the herb's abundant growth, brilliant color, and resemblance to the sun, calendula earned the reputation and the fae energy as a sign of inexhaustible life. It is no wonder, then, that calendula would be the quintes-sential herb for the skin—the largest organ of the entire body.

Solar-Infused Calendula Salve

Calendula can be used in facial toners along with witch hazel, floral waters, and aloe vera gel. The herb is also combined with honey for an effective facial mask. But most often, you'll find calendula as a salve to bring the life force directly to the skin on a daily basis.

INGREDIENTS

3 cups (600 grams) calendula blossoms
I cup (250 milliliters) organic olive oil
¼ cup (60 milliliters) or 2 ounces (56 grams) beeswax
5 to 10 drops lavender essential oil
I ounce (28 grams) lanolin oil
I ounce (28 grams) vegetable glycerin

Harvest the calendula blossoms after the dew dries, before noon, and hull the pet-als. Place the petals into a sterilized, 1-quart (1-liter) glass jar with a tight-sealing lid. Add the organic olive oil. Remove any air pockets by poking gently with the handle of a wooden spoon or a chopstick. Cover with the lid. Place on a sunny windowsill or outdoors on a stone in a southern location. Sing this blessing over the calendula petals:

> *"Blessings on the flowers and roots*
> *Blessings on the stems and fruits*
> *Blessings on the spirit in me*
> *Blessings on this herb's faerie."*

Over the 2 two weeks, visit the calendula oil daily. Observe and feel the warmth in the jar. Turn the contents as you repeat the blessing. After 2 weeks have passed, strain by pressing the oil with a wooden spoon through an unbleached cheesecloth stretched over a metal strainer that has been placed over a bowl.

To prepare the calendula salve, place the beeswax in a jar and put in a double boiler. Once the beeswax is completely melted, slowly add it to the calendula oil, stirring constantly. (A chopstick is a good tool for the stirring.) When blended, stir in the lavender essential oil, lanolin oil, and glycerin. Pour the warm calendula mixture into small, sterile jars.

Yields approximately 20 ounces (560 grams), or about five 4-ounce (113-gram) jars

Note: To ensure that mold is not given birth in either infusion method, it is important that calendula be dry when harvested. Check the infusion for a dark, cloudy formation in the bottom of the jar. *Do not use cloudy oils.* Repeat the process until successful. If you are infusing in a sunny window, use cheesecloth instead of a solid lid to cap the infusion. This allows moisture to evaporate from the oil.

CALENDULA

"I have seen your lover in my dreams and the life that lies before you in my mind's eye. Quiet yourself now, I have much to show you."

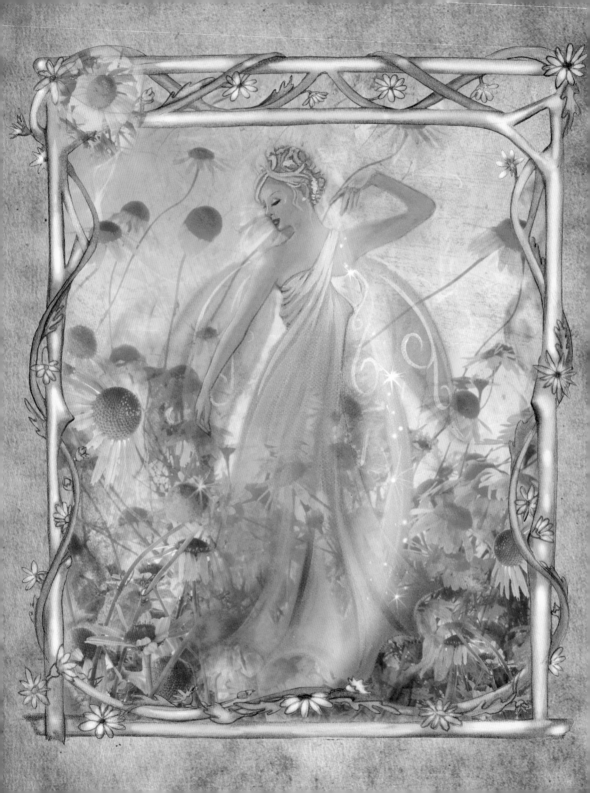

Chamomile

Chamaemelum nobile, Matricaria recutita

Chamaiamelon, Childbed Flower, German Chamomile,
Golden Ball, Ground Apple, Manzanilla, Maythen,
Plants' Physician, Roman Chamomile, White Star

PARTS USED: FLOWERS

Chamomile leaves are feathery, and its fragrant flowers are white, small, and daisy-like with yellow centers. Chamomile is a member of the daisy family. The flowers of German chamomile, *Matricaria recutita*, are used in tea and essential oils. Roman chamomile, *Chamaemelum nobile*, is used in shampoos and cosmetics and as a hair lightener. In ancient earth practices, chamomile was used in prosperity rituals and to aid meditation and was associated with the sun.

Chamomile has been one of the most popular medicinal plants for centuries and is often referred to as childbed flower because it is gentle and used to treat many childhood ailments. Its faerie essence is at once gentle and accessible to all people: it holds no grudges, accepts all, and heals with a soft touch and much compassion. It's kind of like the Buddha of the botanical realm.

Chamomile is an essential natural first-aid home remedy that can be used in a variety of ways. A simple remedy involves placing a warm, moist chamomile tea bag directly on an affected eye for quick relief from conjunctivitis and styes. A couple drops of German-chamomile essential oil mixed with 1 cup (250 milliliters) of flaxseeds and sewn into a rectangle-shaped pouch make a soothing eye pillow. To bring relief to flu aches and pains, combine 2 cups of dried chamomile flowers and 2 quarts (2 liters) of hot water in a medium bowl. Cover your head with a towel, lean over the bowl, and inhale the vapors. Chamomile vapors help destroy germs that cause the flu.

Do not use this steam method if you suffer from cardiovascular disease.

Chamomile tea (1 teaspoon chamomile to 1 cup [250 millileters] water) can be used to gargle, to soothe an upset stomach or psyche, and to fight flu or a cough. Poured into ice trays, chamomile tea ice cubes will cool you down during hot summer days. Chamomile oil (1³/₄ ounces dried flowers or 1 scant cup fresh flowers to 1 pint [500 milliliters] olive oil) will relieve chapped lips. In homeopathy, chamomile is used to treat common children's problems such as stomach cramps, middle ear infection, colic, diarrhea, and teething. For adults, homeopathic use of chamomile has treated gallbladder attacks, menstrual cramps, facial neuralgia, tension headaches, insomnia, asthma, emotional stress, and mood swings. In aromatherapy, chamomile is used as a relaxation agent, particularly with massage and other bodywork. German-chamomile essential oil can also heal burns and relieve joint and muscle pain.

CHAMOMILE

"I know you are looking for a gentle, healing touch. I may be just the faerie you have been searching for. Come have a spot of tea with me and take my hand so that we may know each other."

Chamomile was used throughout ancient Egypt primarily as a nervine and was dedicated to the sun for its profound and gentle healing properties. It is considered to be a guardian spirit in any garden because it heals nearly any plant it grows beside. It is even believed to keep insects at bay. Its effectiveness and ability to bring health to neighboring plants earned chamomile the nickname "plant's physician." Because of its ability to promote general well-being, chamomile is often included in sacred amulets to bring success and/or protection to the wearer.

Chamomile Shower Gel

In this shower gel, chamomile will protect sensitive skin and leave you feeling the compassion inherent in this plant's fae energy. This is perfect gel to use when you are feeling frayed nerves and need comfort and self-acceptance.

INGREDIENTS

$^1/_2$ cup (125 milliliters) rose water
1 cup (250 milliliters) liquid castile soap
  (vegetable-oil based soap)
15 drops chamomile essential oil
8 drops lavender essential oil
8 drops rose geranium essential oil

In a large measuring cup or medium-sized bowl, combine all the ingredients and gently stir to blend, keeping the foam to a minimum.

Yields 12 ounces (375 milliliters) of shower gel

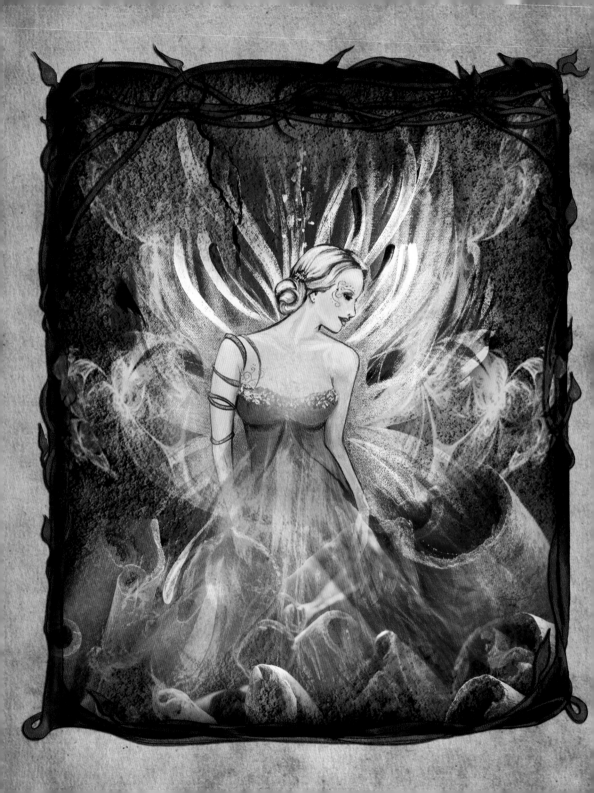

Cinnamon

Cinnamomum zeylanicum

Cassia, Ceylon Cinnamon, Sweet Wood

PARTS USED: INNER BARK

Cinnamon is a small tree with a rust-colored thin trunk, oblong leaves, eggplant-purple pods, red-colored new growth leaves; its flowers, which are arranged in clusters, have a greenish color and a distinct odor. Although this evergreen tree is native to southern India and Sri Lanka, you can grow cinnamon with well-drained sandy loam, plenty of nutrients, and in sun to partial shade. It will grow best in a tropical or humid climate.

Cinnamon has a rich history dating back five thousand years, when Arabs controlled the spice trade and brought cinnamon, from what was known then as the Spice Islands, to sell in Nineveh, Babylon, Egypt, and Rome. Egyptians used cinnamon in their embalming rituals, the Romans used it as a love potion and valued spices as highly as gold, and Nero burned a year's worth of cinnamon in tribute to his dead wife. Even Moses used cinnamon in a holy oil to anoint the ark. By the eleventh century, spices were used in place of currency in many instances, and during the spice wars that followed, control of cinnamon played a vital role.

CINNAMON

"Oh, it is fun being spicy, to bring the heat to the party, and be open to play. Let me dance on your palate and awaken your senses. I'll burn my essence into your world."

Cinnamon's fae energy holds three important ideas together: prosperity, protection, and love. The fae folk tell us to be willing and open to opulence in our life. There is so much good we can do when we can pay our bills and buy the groceries and clothes for the family. It is not selfish to want. A simple way to bring more prosperity into your life is to place three cinnamon sticks in a triangle with the point facing you. Close your eyes and imagine the exact amount of money you will need. Now spin a tale in your head and think about all the many different ways your prosperity can and will positively impact and affect others.

Do not use cinnamon in medicinal amounts if pregnant, and at all times avoid placing cinnamon directly on your skin.

Cinnamon has not only been used for centuries for magickal and emotional purposes, in particular for protection, but it has also been effective medicinally. In Ayurvedic medicine, cinnamon wards off chills in the body and is prescribed to protect the intestines and to work as an antiseptic. Perhaps this warming quality contributed to its reputation as an aphrodisiac.

It's interesting to note that the qualities herbs carry for healing our physical body often correspond with the qualities the herbs carry for healing our emotional or spiritual body. This is most certainly the case with cinnamon. This particular splash will provide warmth that will make you feel protected as well as lend physical protection from colds. It may also help you feel protected in a field of love while you call your lover to you.

Protection Splash

To further enhance the loving of opulence and the protection of your right to roll in the dough, call upon Oshun, the beautiful, lavish Yoruba goddess. Repeat the following phrase three times, in as sultry a tone as you can:

"Oshun, sticky with your honey
Love and money come to me."

INGREDIENTS

1 organic orange
1 organic lemon
1 cup (228 grams) dried lemon verbena
2¼ cups (530 milliliters) vodka
⅔ cup (160 milliliters) orangeflower water
5 drops cinnamon essential oil
5 drops clove essential oil
10 drops orange essential oil
10 drops lemon verbena essential oil

Rinse, dry, and peel the orange and lemon. Place the citrus peels with the dried lemon verbena into a glass jar, then add the vodka. Stir well, cover, and allow to steep for 1 week, shaking occasionally. Strain the mixture into a bowl, discarding the herb and peels. Add the orangeflower water and the essential oils. Stir thoroughly. Place mixture into a glass jar, cover, and store in the refrigerator for 2 months before using.

Yields 48 ounces (1.4 liters)

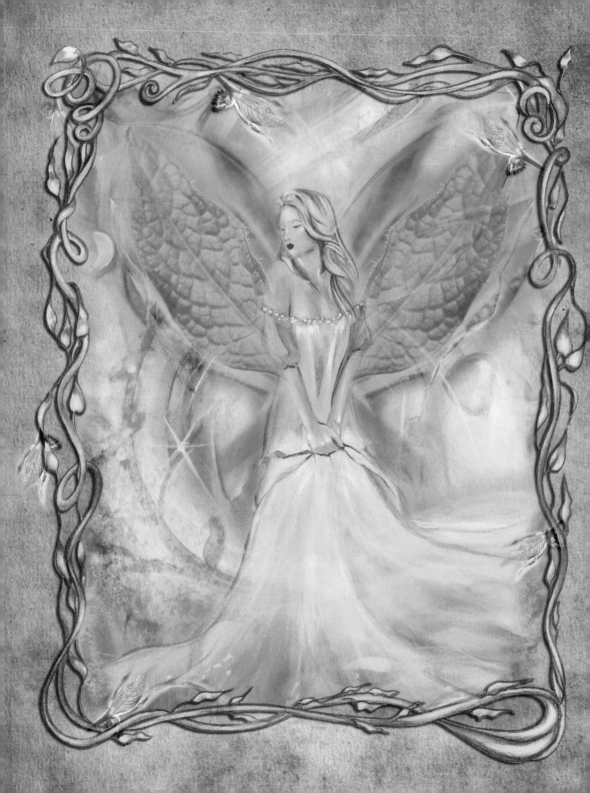

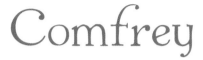

Comfrey

Symphytum officinale

Ass Ear, Blackwort, Boneset, Bruisewort, Coughwort, Gum Plant, Healing Blade, Invisible Vet, Knitback, Knitbone, Slippery Root

PARTS USED: FLOWERING TOPS, LEAVES, STEMS, ROOTS

Comfrey is a perennial herb with a black, turnip-like root and large, hairy, broad leaves. The bell-shaped flowers can be white, cream, yellow, pale blue, purple, or pink, and droop in clusters. The herb can grow to 3 feet in height. Like many herbs, comfrey grows well in full sun, though it can also thrive in shade. It is best to harvest the leaves and flowers in early summer and unearth the root in autumn. Comfrey prefers moist soil and regular watering and will spread quickly through its root system. In the wild, comfrey is found along riverbanks and in marshes.

Comfrey has high levels of protein, calcium, tannins, rosmaric acid, mucilage, and vitamins A, C, and B_{12}. The herb is used in compresses, poultices, teas, tinctures, and ointments. Traditionally, comfrey has been used for protection in travel, perhaps because ancient travelers often journeyed on foot and would need the aid of this herb if they sprained an ankle or broke a bone along the way. It's great for backpackers, too, since very little of the herb is required to make an effective poultice. Take 2 to 4 tablespoons comfrey, dried or fresh, and mix with 1 to 2 teaspoons of water until you achieve a paste. Place a thin cotton cloth over the sprain. Spread a thin layer of poultice over the cloth and leave on for one hour.

When we apply the tenacity and strength of comfrey energy to our endeavors, we can barrel ahead without consideration to our limits. We fool ourselves into being so tough that we can't feel the pain of life's setbacks. We must remember to recognize the time for rest, lest our bodies give us a "break." Respect the skeletal structure, says comfrey. Take yourself lightly, adapt with the changes, grow slowly, don't isolate yourself, but enjoy the course of unfolding manifestation. Define where you stand, but be willing to bend to the forge fires when necessary.

Comfrey is associated with the astrological sign of Capricorn. The fae essence of this herb centers around the improbable ability to achieve the impossible through hard work and relentless dedication. It is interesting to note that the sign of Capricorn is related to the skeletal structure, and since the first century comfrey has been used to promote the healing of bruises, sprains, and broken bones. Of course, faerie energy would be incomplete without some sort of humor, and in the case of Capricorns, they begin life with a grave attitude and, with age, learn not to take themselves so seriously and eventually to lighten up a great deal. Capricorn is ruled by Saturn, the God of Time, and is also associated to Hephaestus, the Greek God of the Forge and Smith Crafting. A smith crafter takes hard metal and applies fire to bend it to create tools and works of art. Thus, the healing message of comfrey is to learn the delicate balance between establishing structure and being flexible enough to change with the times.

COMFREY

"Can I come with you? I'm great help when you fall and can ease you back into life with my wit. I'm not as shy as I look and am a comfort when you are injured. My pleasure comes from reminding you to play and that, at times, it is also productive to enjoy this gift of life we share."

Comfy Comfrey Salve

This is an excellent salve to soothe the burning pain and itching from razor burn. It is for external use only, but is quite effective on sensitive areas of the skin. As you make this salve, make a promise to take yourself more lightly. Learn to laugh at your mistakes and accept your imperfections as perfectly human. Hephaestus, the divine energy associated with this herb, was crippled and yet the most talented of all the gods on Olympus. He could take anything—garbage or the most precious metal—and make something useful and beautiful. He learned to make the best of his talents and let everything else just slide off his back. Enjoy what you do well and allow this soothing salve to bring you the healing relief you so deserve.

Don't use this salve on cuts deeper than $^1/_4$-inch if the wound is bleeding profusely, or if the wound was caused by a splinter, other foreign object, or an animal bite.

INGREDIENTS

$1^1/_2$ cups (375 milliliters) water
$^1/_3$ cup (76 grams) dried comfrey leaves
$1^1/_2$ tablespoons coconut oil
$^1/_4$ cup (55 grams) beeswax, softened
20 drops lavender essential oil

Bring the water to a boil in a saucepan. Turn off the heat, add the comfrey, and cover with a lid. Allow the infusion to sit for 2 hours. Strain the liquid and discard the comfrey. (You can add it to your compost heap, or just sprinkle in your garden or lawn.) Pour 1 cup (250 milliliters) of the comfrey infusion into a saucepan over low heat. Add the oil. Shave or cut the beeswax into small chunks and slowly add it to the infusion. Heat until the beeswax is melted, then remove from the heat and add the lavender oil. Pour the salve into sterilized containers. Store the salve in a cool, dark place, and use it within one year.

Yields approximately three 4-ounce (113-gram) jars

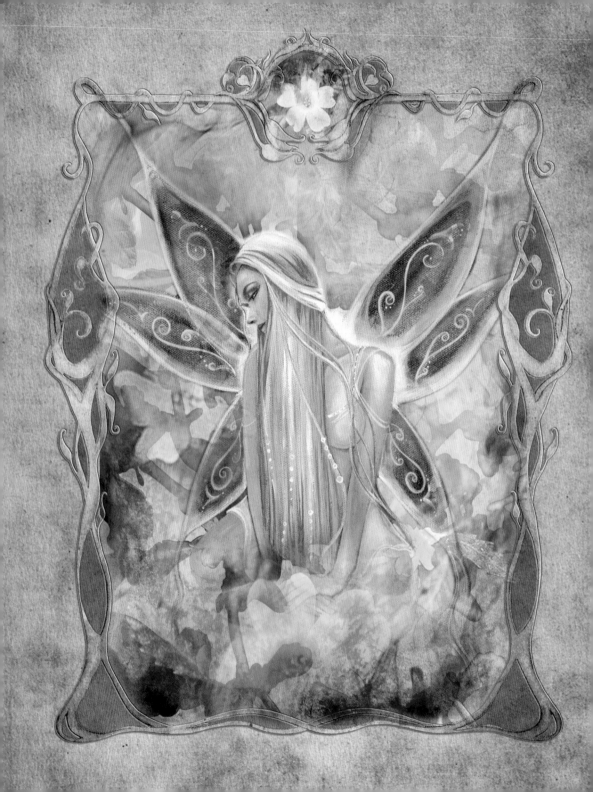

Damiana

Turnera aphrodisiaca

Herba de la Pastora, Mexican Damiana, Old Woman's Broom

PARTS USED: LEAVES

A small shrub, damiana has leaves that are smooth and pale green on the upper side. The yellow flowers blossom in early to late summer and are followed by fruits that taste similar to figs. The leaves and stems of the damiana plant are gathered at the time of flowering. Damiana has a strong aromatic herbal scent slightly reminiscent of chamomile. It thrives in any good soil if given a sunny location. It should be watered freely from spring to fall, and sparingly in winter.

Of all the things this little plant can do, damiana is best known as an aphrodisiac and raises sexual desire in men and women. Spanish missionaries first recorded that native Mexicans drank damiana tea mixed with sugar for its ability to enhance lovemaking.

When using damiana for its aphrodisiac qualities, try pairing with Freya, the Norse Goddess of Sensual Love and War. Usually depicted as a spectacular strawberry blond with stunning blue eyes, Freya was legendary for her unbridled sexuality and far surpassed any other exploits of the world's pantheons of Goddesses of Love or Beauty.

Outside of the bedroom, Freya still held considerable power. She had the right to claim half the souls of the bravest warriors who died in battle. Visiting the battlefield, she gathered fallen soldiers and took them back with her to Valhalla, to live in perpetual rest and recreation. When Freya and the Valkyries rode forth on their missions, their armor caused the eerily beautiful flickering light that we know as the Aurora Borealis, or Northern Lights. She wore a falcon cloak and rode in a chariot drawn by two large cats. Her magickal necklace of amber and rubies, made by dwarves, was called a "brisling" or "brisingamen," and it made her irresistible. Freya's passions remind us to explore and acknowledge all of our emotions, longings, and traits. Since Friday was named after the Goddess Freya, try making your damiana liqueur on Friday to truly bring out the Freya in you.

In each one of us exists a powerfully sensual being. When she turns on her sex appeal, like Freya, none can resist her. Her passion cannot be contained—it knows no limits or boundaries and is free from all shame or condemnation. For not only does she possess alluring sensuality, but she is also fierce and commanding. She is Divine. She is Deity. She is your Sacred Slut—your Holy Whore and you've ignored her for far too long. Are you cringing? Remember, if it were not for her lustful energy, her desire to couple, humanity would not exist. She is holy to all who live. And she's waiting for you to take her out of the darkness and bring her to the light—to put her on her rightful pedestal where she can be admired and adored.

Damiana Liqueur

INGREDIENTS

2/3 cup (155 grams) crumbled damiana leaves and stems

2 tablespoons anise liquer

2 tablespoons ground cardamom

2 tablespoons ground cinnamon

1 tablespoon ground ginger

3 cups (750 milliliters) brandy

2 tablespoons vanilla extract

3/4 cup (165 grams) honey

3/4 cup (165 grams) black cherry concentrate

1 tablespoon rose water

As you drop the damiana flowers into the bottle imagine that you are at the end of a long hallway. At the opposite end is a door. Walk slowly toward the door, knowing that the essence, the embodiment of *your* sexuality, is on the other side, calling you. Notice what hangs on the walls of the halls as you walk to the door. Finally, turn the handle and open the door.

There she is. What does she look like? What does her room look like? Does she have a name? Does she say anything to you? Speak her name or anything about her into the bottle. Add the other herbs and pour the brandy on top. Allow it to steep for 2 weeks.

During the week, think of your sacred, sexual being often. Befriend her. Know that this entrantress is a truly sacred aspect of your goddess self. Two weeks later, on a Friday, strain out the herbs through muslin. Hold the honey and imagine it as an elixir from Freya's necklace of desire. As you pour the amber liquid

DAMIANA

"My sensuality and seductive ways attract all mortals and make me the perfect faerie for grown-up play."

into the brandy, imagine that Freya, a consciousness that for centuries has represented the powerful Goddess of Sensuality, is embracing your unique expression of sexuality and passion. Stir well. Pour in the black sherry currant and rose water next and visualize yourself as attracting passion and purity. Now go and have some fun.

Yields approximately 1 quart (1 liter)

Note: You can substitute the brandy for vodka. If you have difficulty finding black cherry concentrate, then you can substitute another berry or even peach concentrate.

The inspiration for this ritual came from Nila Keith, who, with Jamie, co-led a group of sultry women on this meditation while at a goddess retreat in Kadavu, Fiji. Let's just say it was quite effective.

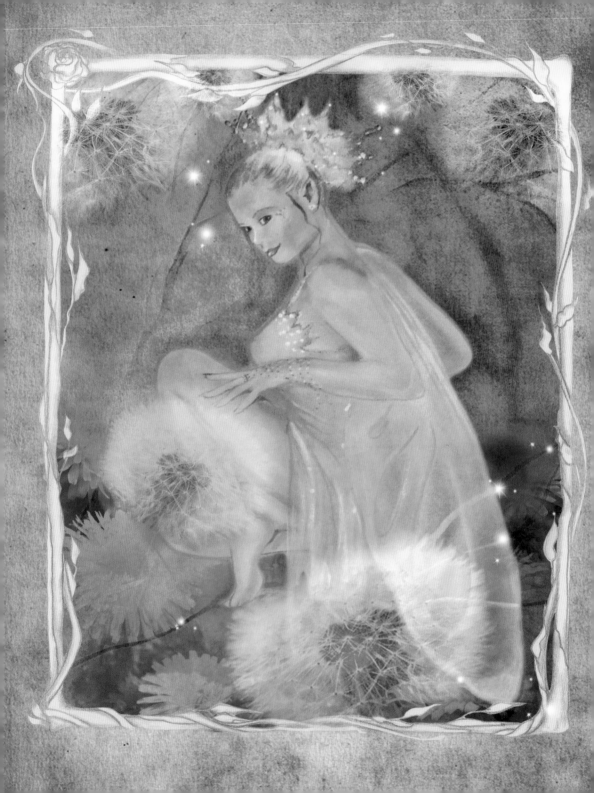

Dandelion

Taraxacum officinale

Blow Balls, Dent de Lion, Goat's Beard, Lion's Tooth, Peasant's Cloak,
Pee-a-Bed, Priest's Crown, Swine Snout, Wild Chicory

PARTS USED: LEAVES, ROOTS, STEMS

Dandelion leaves are jagged lobes that point back toward the stem. The flowers are long and yellow and have a honey scent.

Dandelion is a very powerful diuretic. It is one of the best natural sources of potassium as well as vitamin A, calcium, and iron. It has been used to remedy muscular rheumatism and jaundice. The juice of dandelion has been used to treat diabetes and liver disease. It is one of the best herbs for building blood and treating anemia: simply eat the dandelion greens as your salad. If used in early pregnancy, dandelion can relieve nausea and indigestion. Ten to 20 drops of dandelion root tincture in 1 cup (250 milliliters) of water with meals and before bed can help alleviate water retention. You can use the leaves in an herbal bath or facial steam. The flowers can be used to obtain a yellow dye for wools, or if you use the entire plant, you will get a magenta color.

Ever since we were children, we turned to the dandelion to wish us to a new place. We'd pluck the flower near its base and hold that little puffball inches from our mouth. We'd close our eyes and dream of a better place. Sometimes we'd use our inner vision to see it, smell it, hear it, taste it, feel it. Then we'd take a deep breath and blow, sending the mini seeds flying in all directions to fall somewhere out there, to plant themselves and manifest our dreams. And if we could just get every last seed off the flower head, we trusted our dream would come true. It's no wonder this plant is associated with the astrological sign of Sagittarius, the quintessential gypsy, trusting, life seeker.

Dandelion Meditation

Go out to your garden or a nearby park for a meditation to reconnect, remember, and reunite with nature and the fae essence of dandelion and you. Take a dandelion flower—as a plant, a tincture, a tea, or greens. Or seek the dandelion as you journey to your destination—whether you're driving to a park or walking out through your back woods or taking the elevator to the top of your building where you can feel the wind blow.

Take three deep breaths as you arrive. Close your eyes and get comfy. Drop into your sadness, your anger, your fear. Pack all those heavy feelings into a ball. Imagine that a bright, extremely hot fire ignites below the ball. The ball bursts into flames. Sparks of fire spin off from the explosion, and like fireflies, dance around you playfully, rejoicing to be freed of negativity. Watch as they come together as a ball of light that dances on the air in front of you.

The ball of light bounces away from you. Follow it along until you come to the thickest, deepest part of the unknown where the ancient trees grow, towering to brush against the sky. Imagine the twinkling of lights scattered through the shadows. Feel the tingle in your toes as you realize you have entered the magickal realm of unthinking, unbound energy where there is no future, no past. In this place, the world between the worlds, there is only the present. Here in the world of illumination, anything is possible.

DANDELION

"I am the complete package for your health, from food to medicine to magick wishes. I'd be happy to get to know you, but first, let's despense with the 'weed' title you've given me, shall we? I feel so misunderstood."

Imagine the ball of light dancing in front of you. See a pool. Bend down and look at your reflection in this luminescent place. What is that you see? Do you see love and kindness looking back? See if you can catch that moment when the flicker of faerie spirit became you: the freed, enchanted you.

Feel the quietness beyond the questions and answers. This stillness is the faerie energy that sustains and empowers you and your unique expression. This is the faerie's message in meditation: Find yourself. Find the juicy, ripe, burgeoning part of you and give it all your energy. Feed it, like you would nurture a child. Pour your attention into your individual perspective, your unique expression, for this is your greatest gift to the world.

You can either try this meditation with a simple dandelion tea (1 tablespoon herb to 1 cup [250 milliliters] water) or incorporate the visualization with this salad.

Divine Dandelion Salad

INGREDIENTS

1½ cups (340 grams) dandelion
    greens, chopped
¼ cup (55 grams) cheese
½ cup (113 grams) caramelized pecans
¼ cup (55 grams) grape tomatoes
1 soft persimmon, sliced

DRESSING

¼ cup (60 milliliters) balsamic vinegar
1 teaspoon Dijon mustard
1 teaspoon sugar
½ teaspoon salt
½ teaspoon pepper
1 clove garlic, pressed
½ cup (113 grams) extra virgin olive oil

Mix together the salad ingredients. In a small stainless steel or glass bowl, whisk together the vinegar, mustard, sugar, salt, pepper, and garlic until the sugar and salt are dissolved. While continuing to whisk, add the olive oil in a thin, steady stream. Pour the vinaigrette onto the salad. Toss well.

Serves 4 to 6

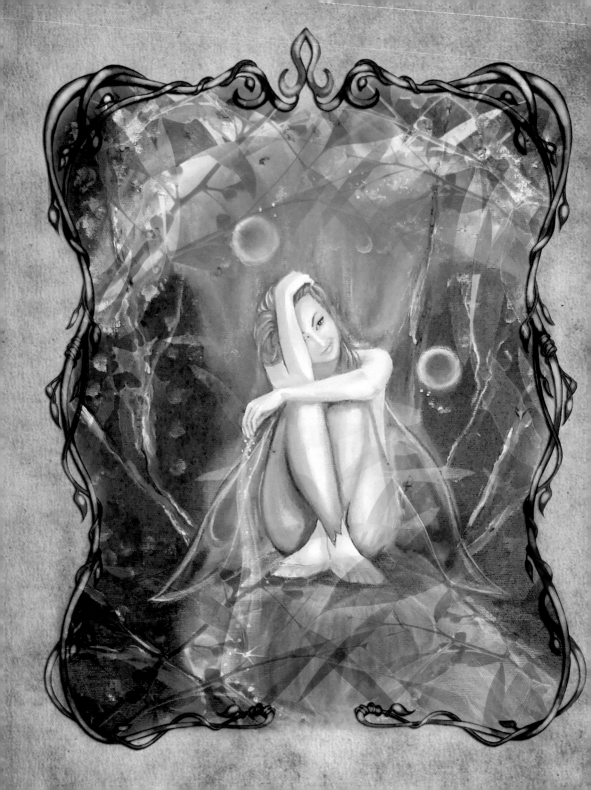

Eucalyptus

Eucalyptus (various species)

Blue Gum, Fever Tree

PARTS USED: LEAVES

There are many varieties of eucalyptus trees and even shrubs. The trees can be categorized as forest, woodland, mallet, mallee, or marlock. The forest trees are single-stemmed and have a crown forming a minor proportion of the whole tree height. Woodland trees are single-stemmed, although they may branch at a short distance above ground level. The smooth bark of mallets often has a satiny sheen and may be white, cream, gray, green, or copper. Mallees are multi-stemmed and can grow so low they are sometimes considered a shrub. Marlocks are short, erect, thin-stemmed trees.

Eucalyptus is best known for relieving bronchial and nasal congestion and fighting infections. It helps us breathe. Its faerie essence relates to our capacity to take in life to its fullest. It relates to the ability and willingness to be overjoyed. The essential oil is found in disinfectants, insect repellant, and products that provide relief from sinus problems and sore muscles. Rubbing the essential oil on

EUCALYPTUS

"Welcome to my world, where all is not as it seems. Let me shower you with new beginnings when all you see is the end. Together we can fly closer to where true harmony lies."

fingernails can strengthen them. Eucalyptus essential oil can also be added to bath water to combat flu or mixed into a bowl of warm water and inhaled for relief from blocked sinuses. If you don't have the time or inclination to try the recipe below, you can still tap into the power of eucalyptus by making a simple facial steam that will help remove you from the irritation of another and alleviate suffering from sinus problems or breathing issues. Fill a bowl with at least 1 quart (1 liter) of steaming water. Add 5 to 10 drops of eucalyptus essential oil. Cover your head with a cloth and lean over the bowl. Repeat the chant opposite. Breathe deeply and allow the words to wash over you until you believe them.

All-Natural Carpet Cleaner

Eucalyptus is a favorite ingredient for herbal cleansers. This simple all-purpose carpet cleaner will disinfect and deodorize, as well as repel fleas, nits, and worm eggs. You can sprinkle it on your rug or carpeting before vacuuming regularly or even add $1/4$ cup (60 milliliters) solution to $3^1/_2$ gallons (14 liters) water to steam cleaners.

As you move your furniture preparing for a deep cleansing, this cleanser will have the dual purpose of allowing you to release some of the stale energy that has built up not only in your home but in your psyche as well.

Eucalyptus is associated with Pluto, the God of the Underworld, in charge of rebirth, as in the phoenix rising from the ashes. The God of the Underworld seems at first to be an enemy, knocking us down, taking away all that we hold dear. In fact, he is strengthening us, asking us to continually renew ourselves, to evolve and become more each day than we were the day before. Only in this constant recycling and growing can we find the freedom that Pluto is nudging us toward.

Eucalyptus is also connected to the moon, the planetary orb that rules over our emotions. As this herb heals sinus problems, it is interesting to note that sinusitis is often related to being annoyed by someone close to you. Perhaps she is pushing your buttons as Pluto is asking you to allow parts of yourself to die so that you can be regenerated, fresh, and new. It is said that those who annoy us the most are our best teachers. They are simply mirroring something we have not completely accepted about ourselves. As you clean the foundation of your home, consider that you are also cleaning the foundation of your inner spirit. Repeat this chant either aloud or quietly to yourself, being careful to keep your eyes closed.

> *"All is well and harmonious in my world.*
> *Angels surround me wherever I go.*
> *I am at peace with all that I see and hear.*
> *All is well and harmonious in my world."*

INGREDIENTS

I quart (900 grams) borax
2 tablespoons baking soda
25 drops eucalyptus essential oil
25 drops lavender essential oil
25 drops rosemary essential oil

Mix all the ingredients together.

Yields just over I quart (900 grams)

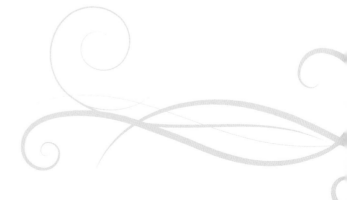

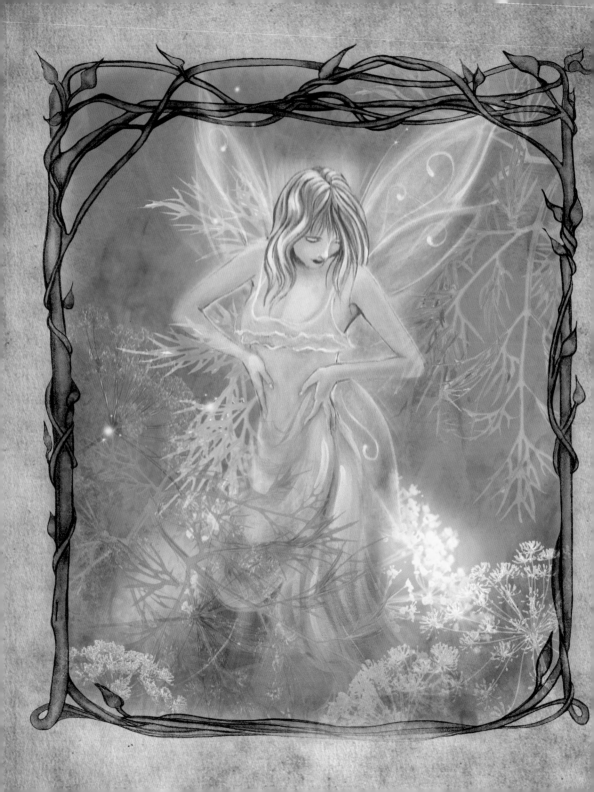

fennel

Foeniculum vulgare

Fenkel, Sweet Fennel

PARTS USED: FRESH STEMS, SEEDS, LEAVES, ROOTS

Fennel is a licorice-flavored herb with feathery plumes of grass-green foliage and stunning umbrella-shaped yellow flowers. It prefers full sun, warm temperature, and well-drained, humus-rich soil.

Fennel has been used from Jamaica to China to Africa to treat gastric ailments, obesity, cramps, rheumatism, and diabetes. It improves memory, works as a laxative, soothes the digestive system, increases breast milk production, and helps fight infection. Seeds ground to a powder can deter fleas. You can also chew fennel seeds found in the wild, if you are certain the area has not been sprayed with chemicals, to alleviate stomach pains or indigestion or to freshen the breath.

The ancient ones believed taking fennel would bestow long life, courage to face danger, wisdom in the face of adversity, and sexual virility and fertility. As an Herb of Protection, fennel was traditionally gathered on Midsummer's Eve and hung over portals to guard loved ones inside. This custom was usually done to protect from the fae folk, who were experienced tricksters without heed for convention. Today, as we welcome the faeries into our lives, we find that fennel can serve as a tool to open ourselves to other realms, to right brain thinking and fields of possibilities. In fact, Saxons valued fennel for its ability to deepen the meditation experience. For centuries until the present time, fennel has come highly recommended for those fasting for either spiritual reasons or to cleanse the body of toxins. During a fast, fennel will alleviate hunger pangs, calm the stomach, and increase clairvoyance.

In Kabbalism, fennel is associated with the Sphere of Hod, found in the sacred Tree of Life. The Sphere of Hod contains the energy of staying clear-minded and open, despite the obstacles found in life. In other words, the faerie energy of this plant teaches us to quite literally go with the flow, whether physically, through its work as a digestive aid, or spiritually, through the guidance it offers in meditation. When caught in emotional drama, the best option is to go to trust, riding atop the intensity and stories, rather than getting mired in the muck and forcing solutions.

Life is a process of unfolding. You are never going to figure it out. The answers will reveal themselves to you when you are ready to hear the answers.

FENNEL

"On this path of new discovery I will take you deeper, bring you protection, and help you open your third eye to another dimension."

Interestingly, fennel is also associated with Mercury, the god and plant that governs communication and travel. Healthy communication and the utmost enjoyment of traveling are matters of proper flow and allowing the energy to move where it is needed. The concept of using a talking stick comes to mind. Indeed, the symbol of Mercury is the wand or caduceus, the symbol of health and healing.

Free Spirit Salad

As you share this meal with friends or family, practice communicating with a talking stick or simply imagine a talking stick or the Sphere of Hod moving from person to person as the energy moves. Simply bear witness as the need to offer communication rises in each person in perfect harmony.

INGREDIENTS

1 medium fennel bulb (about 1 pound, or 450 grams),
   peeled, leaves discarded, and cut into thin strips
1 pint (455 grams) mini sweet bell peppers, julienned
$1/4$ cup (55 grams) sun-dried tomatoes
$1/4$ cup (60 milliliters) extra virgin olive oil
$1/2$ cup (120 milliliters) balsamic vinegar
2 teaspoons cracked black pepper
$1/8$ cup (28 grams) grated Asiago cheese

Toss the fennel, bell peppers, and tomatoes in a bowl. In a small bowl, whisk the oil, vinegar, and pepper. Pour over the salad and mix well to coat. Cover and refrigerate the salad for 1 hour. Sprinkle the cheese over the salad before serving.

Serves 4 to 6

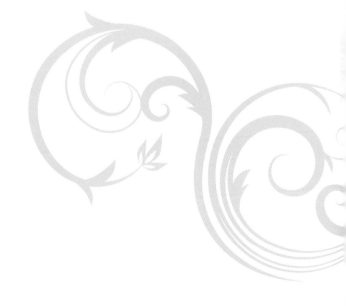

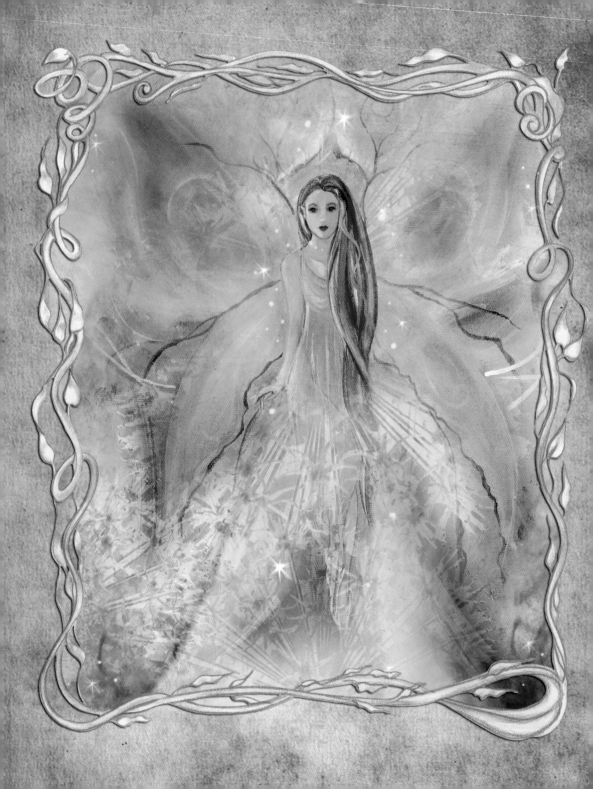

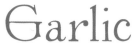

Garlic

Allium sativum

Clove Garlic, Poor Man's Treacle, Stinking Rose

PARTS USED: CLOVES, LEAVES, FLOWERS

Garlic prefers warm climates, full sun, composted soil, and regular watering. Plant whole bulbs in winter after the ground has thawed, and harvest in mid-September. It is also a good idea to plant your garlic near roses to keep the aphids away.

Both Ayurvedic and Chinese medicine revere garlic's healing properties. Its main curative powers fight bacterial and fungal infections, lower high blood pressure and cholesterol levels, and aid the digestive system. Garlic is a strong antiseptic and works wonderfully on mucous membranes. At the onset of a common cold or flu, swallowing a clove of garlic has been effective in preventing the illness from taking hold in the body. It can also be used to treat disorders of the blood and lungs, including tuberculosis, while some reports have shown that it may prevent cancer. Garlic is used to protect the body and hair from parasites and helps with asthma, whooping cough, goiter, arthritis, sciatica, and rheumatism. Garlic is often combined with mullein, and sometimes willow, to relieve earaches.

In esoteric practices, garlic is used for protection and banishing. It has been associated with Mars, Hecate, Kali Maa, the moon, and the Triple Goddess.

Magical Protection Besom

Often around springtime we get the feeling that we're carrying around too much stuff. We do our purge or spring cleaning, clearing out closets, reorganizing attics and basements, washing the windows. But what about getting rid of all our emotional baggage? A besom is a magickal tool used to ritually "sweep out the old." You can either decorate a new broom or make your own besom from scratch. It is a tradition for modern magickal practitioners to buy a new broom or make a besom whenever they move into a new home.

To make your own besom, gather a large fallen tree branch, 1 to 2 inches in diameter, for the handle. Be sure to use a fallen branch—do not use a freshly cut branch to make your besom. Knowing the kind of tree your branch comes from is helpful, because you can call on the specific energy of that tree during the ritual. For example, branches from eucalyptus, hawthorn, bay laurel, or birch, can be referenced in this book for the kind of energy they carry. Alternatively, ash is also an important tree, one of the nine sacred trees, also known as the Tree of Life or the Tree of Knowledge.

For the broom's bristles, gather long-stemmed herbs, such as lavender, bay laurel, eucalyptus, hay, wheat, or straw. Overlap the bristles about 6 inches from the end of the handle, making sure they evenly cover its circumference. Approximately 3 inches from the top of the bristles, tightly bind the bundle to your handle with twine. Then tie 3 bulbs of garlic to the broom.

Add a colored ribbon to your besom. Choose the color with a specific intent, for example, red or pink for love, blue for peace, green or gold for abundance, yellow for friendship, orange for spirituality. You can also add bells to the ties holding the herbs to the handle to represent the calling in of new ideas. Glue or tie anything else to the besom that has meaning to you, such as seashells, beads, bird feathers, or crystals, in order to strengthen your intention and hide any construction flaws.

To bless your new besom, use symbols from each of the four directions: east–air, west–water, south–fire, north–earth. For example, you can waft incense smoke or an embering sage stick, also known as a smudge stick, around your broom, sprinkle purified water, essential oils, or seawater over the besom, pass the besom (not too close) to the flame of a candle, and sprinkle with salt.

Take your besom and either choose a room in your home or go outside into your yard for this ritual. If indoors, begin sweeping the floor while visualizing your emotional baggage as dust and dirt that's obscuring a gleaming, polished hardwood floor. If outdoors, sweep the ground as you imagine the clods of earth and leaf litter making way for rich loamy soil waiting to be cultivated. As you sweep, begin chanting:

"I infuse this besom with the will of my desire,
Invoking the love and protection of my pixie fire.
I let go and release what I no longer want to keep,
Welcoming blessings, wealth, and the light each time that I sweep."

Visualize all the negative, stale energy leaving your home and see the room bathed in warmth and light that will not only protect you but also help you focus on the blessings and good fortune you intend to attract. In your mind's eye, see all the people you will welcome into your bright, airy home, and see all the new herbs, plants, trees, and animals your lovingly tended garden will attract and support.

GARLIC

"When working with me, you will clean away the old and banish what is not working. From there we can create a space for new growth and rebirth. My healing can be felt from the heart both physically and emotionally."

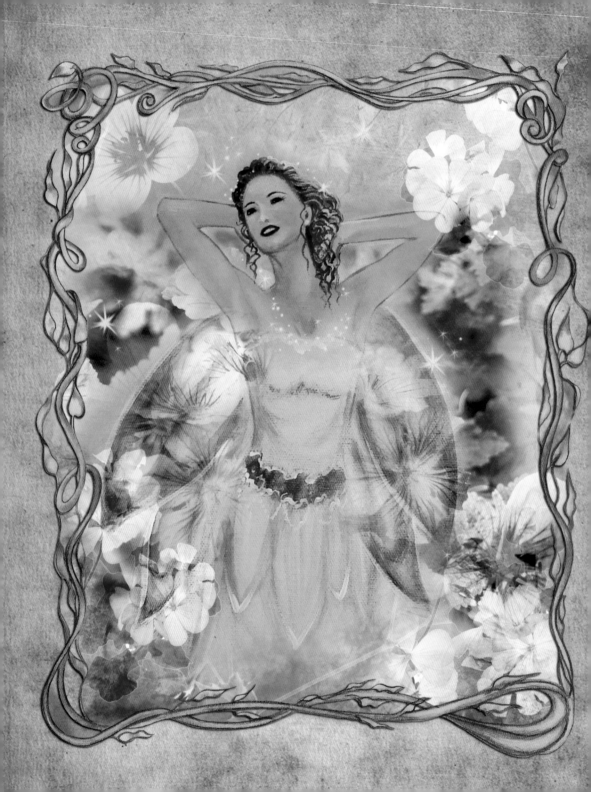

Geranium

Pelargonium (various species)

Cranesbill, Storksbill

PARTS USED: LEAVES, FLOWERS

Geranium is a genus of 422 species of flowering annual, biennial, and perennial plants with flowers ranging in color from red, blue, and purple to vibrant pinks and white. Usually, geraniums prefer a sunny location and need a lot of space to grow. Rose geranium can root from a cutting by either placing it directly in the soil or putting the cutting in water first.

The word *geranium* comes from the Greek word *geranos*, meaning "crane." According to native traditions, cranes represent self-reflection and the necessary action of going inward. Geranium also resonates with Venus (love), Isis (feminine power), Gaia (Earth Mother energy), Eros (love), Hecate (mystery), Venus (love), Mars (assertiveness), and the Horned One (fertility). Geranium is associated with the astrological sign of Libra (balance). Combining all these symbols, we find that geranium holds in balance and harmony female and male power, invoking love and bringing about fertility. It accomplishes this through the crane's grace and mystery, all the while looking good doing it, as Libras also prize aesthetics. The faerie essence of this herb attracts fertility, balance, harmony, protection, and love.

GERANIUM

"What a lovely day to begin living with an open heart. I am delicate and dewy in the morning, smelling fresh and sweet. So just sit with me and enjoy the view. Breathe deeply the spirit of life."

Rose geranium (the common name for various species and cultivars, including *Pelargonium capitatum* and *Pelargonium graveolens*) has citrus and rose scents that provide a unique combination. An essential oil made from this plant can be rubbed on the wrists to ease menstrual cramps, depression, menopausal symptoms, hormonal imbalances, and fluid retention. Rose geranium works as a tonic on your central nervous system. Geranium has a profound ability to clean and heal all kinds of wounds. When added to skin lotions, creams, or salves, rose geranium has been known to aid acne, eczema, and inflamed and infected wounds, and even to delay wrinkles.

Rose geranium carries the energy to grant the ability to look at your feelings and opinions with an open heart and calm demeanor. It can help you stay alert and conscious to all of life. It can remind you to count your blessings, however small or inconsequential they may seem compared to your obstacles.

Rose Geranium Herbal Deodorant

This focus on the blessings will bring you back to the fact that you are the cocreator in your life. Everything that is going on in your life, you created because at the time, it served your need. Perhaps what you created no longer works or you've outgrown it. It's okay to let go. Everything you put into your body serves its purpose, and the excess is flushed our through the lymphatic system, particularly through our underarms. Release without judgment and focus on the blessings, says rose geranium.

INGREDIENTS

2 teaspoons zinc oxide powder

$^1/_2$ cup (120 milliliters) witch hazel

2 teaspoons aloe vera juice

30 drops rose geranium essential oil

In a small bowl, stir the zinc oxide powder into the witch hazel. Add the aloe vera juice and rose geranium essential oil. Pour into a dark glass spray bottle.

Yields 8 ounces (250 milliliters)

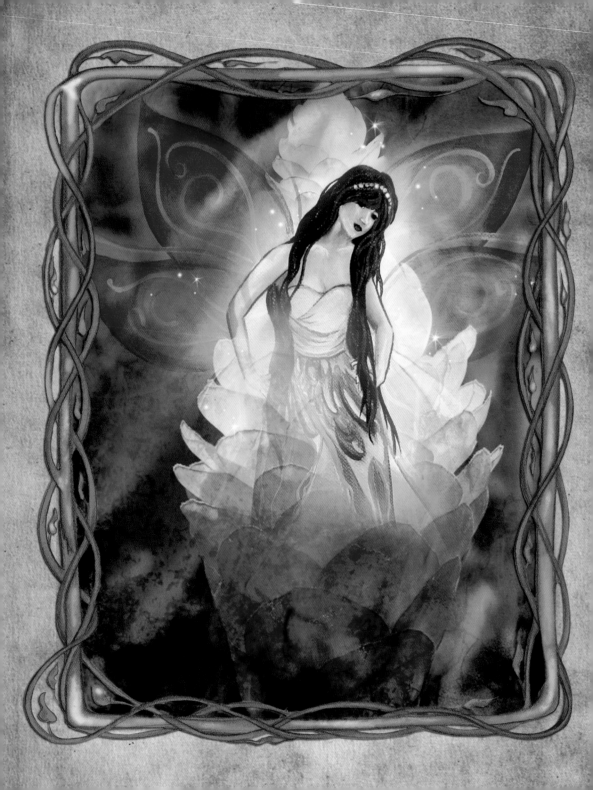

Ginger

Zingiber officinale

African Ginger, Black Ginger, Canton Ginger, Jamaican Ginger, True Ginger

PARTS USED: ROOTS, LEAVES

Ginger is a perennial root that creeps and increases underground. In the spring it sends up from its roots a green reed, like a stalk, 2 feet high, with long, narrow, ribbed green leaves and white, yellowish green, fuchsia, or orange-yellow flowers. Ginger's roots spread far and wide and are difficult to uproot once they have established themselves. It prefers fertile soil and plenty of watering.

Ginger has been used in Chinese and Ayurvedic medicine for centuries. Ginger has a warming quality that aids digestive problems, stimulates circulation, promotes sweating, reducing fevers, relieves colds, and alleviates pain. It inhibits blood clotting and is believed to prevent arteriosclerosis. Ginger is also believed to fight against cancer. Ginger root is known to have antioxidant effects; it contains compounds that protect cells from excess free radicals, which can trigger all kinds of cell mutations that can lead to cancer. Ginger has also been proven to inhibit the growth of certain fungi that produce potent carcinogens. Ginger is a general tonic for nerves as well as the digestive organs; its primary healing abilities are to quell motion sickness and prevent indigestion. The faerie essence of this herb assists us in the ability to process life—to use the best of what is given to us and let go of the rest.

Those with gallstones should consult a health practitioner before using ginger.

Ginger Tea

The most common way to ingest ginger is in tea form. Ginger tea (2 teaspoons dried or 1 teaspoon fresh ginger to 1 cup [250 milliliters] boiling water, then strain) will relieve gastrointestinal and menstrual cramps. Or you can add ¹/₂ teaspoon clove blossoms and 1 teaspoon chamomile flowers to ¹/₂ teaspoon ginger root to relieve nausea and vomiting and stimulate saliva flow and digestive activity. The warmth that ginger tea brings to the body makes it excellent for chasing away chills and colds. You can choose to sweeten the tea with stevia, agave, honey, or lemon. You can also soak a towel in the tea and apply to sore muscles or a congested chest for relief.

Ginger fights nausea, which is related to the rejection of life's natural flow. Nausea comes on when we fear the new and unfamiliar. If life were predictable, there would be no point in living. This earth experience is about reaching, always reaching for more— to discover what is around the next bend. To tap into the faerie energy of this herb, we need to combat our fear of the mysterious with the trust that everything is moving along smoothly. This is important for those times when life's twisty turns seem to make no sense at all.

GINGER

"Do not fear the unpredictable, for I am with you. I can guide you through new experiences and help you float in trust while taming your distressed tummy. I may be spicy, but I'm also sweet. Just as life. Just as this journey."

Ginger will help you face the unknown with its warming qualities. According to ancient medicinal practices, such as Ayurveda, when our digestive system is healthy, we can expect to feel an overall health and harmony in our body, including our physical as well as our emotional or spiritual body. In fact, serotonin, the natural chemical that helps us feel good, is produced in the gut: so a happy gut equals a happy person. Draw upon the healing qualities of ginger to expect positive, joyful experiences on this strange journey called Life.

Exotic Tofu

INGREDIENTS

2 blocks extra-firm tofu
$^1/_2$ cup (125 milliliters) soy sauce
$^1/_2$ cup (125 milliliters) balsamic vinegar
$^1/_4$ cup (60 milliliters) water
2 tablespoons finely chopped ginger root
1 cup (250 milliliters) peanut sauce
$1^1/_2$ tablespoons Bragg Liquid Aminos
$^1/_2$ cup (113 grams) shredded unsweetened coconut
$^1/_2$ cup (113 grams) finely chopped macadamia nuts
2 tablespoons sesame oil

Slice the tofu on a diagonal. Then slice again, lengthwise, to form triangles. Squeeze excess water from the tofu by gently pressing down with a paper towel or cloth napkin. Place heavy dishes on top of the tofu to compress and leave for at least 4 hours, or overnight.

Mix together the soy sauce, balsamic vinegar, water, and ginger root. Add the peanut sauce. Place the compressed tofu triangles in a shallow baking dish and drizzle the liquid aminos over the tofu. Pour three-quarters of the ginger-peanut mixture over the tofu and marinate for 45 minutes.

Preheat the oven to 375°F (190°C). Combine the coconut and macadamia nuts. Heat the sesame oil into large skillet over medium heat. Dip one side of each tofu triangle into the coconut/macadamia nut mixture. Place in the skillet and cook until browned, approximately 4 to 6 minutes. Return the cooked tofu to the baking dish. Drizzle with the remaining ginger-peanut sauce and bake for 25 to 30 minutes, or until heated through.

Serves 10 to 12

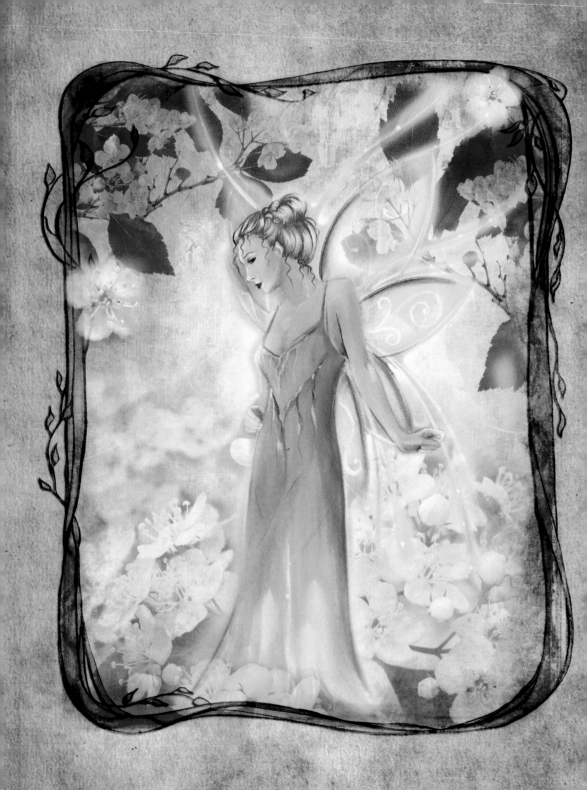

hawthorn

Crataegus (various species)

Bread and Cheese Tree, Faeriethorn, Halves, Huath, Ladies' Meat,
May Blossom, May Tree, Quick, Tree of Chastity, White Thorn

PARTS USED: BERRIES, WOOD, BRANCHES, SEEDS, FLOWERS

hawthorn is a tree or shrub with thorny branches and small, white pinkish flowers that are fragrant and grow in clusters. The bark is smooth gray in young individuals, developing shallow long fissures with narrow ridges in older trees. The tree bears small red, hard fruits called haws. The trees become quite gnarled over time and live to a ripe old age. Hawthorn likes full sun, light watering, and well-drained soil without too much amendment. Hawthorn grows wild in wastelands, heaths, hedges, and woods of temperate regions throughout the Northern Hemisphere.

The name hawthorn is derived from a Greek word meaning "strength." Hawthorn is the quintessential faerie tree. Its faerie essence is the guardian, the marker to the faerie realm. It is one of the faerie tree triad of Celtic lore of "Oak, Ash, and Thorne." Falling asleep under the hawthorn tree during the month of May is said to bring a faerie tryst, a time in faerieland. However long you stay is up to you. But it's wise to remember that time moves differently in fae, whether you spell it fey, faerie, or fairy—it's always the same, and always different. The light filters in a unique way in the slant that is the fae realm. It is a parallel universe with a set of laws and social concepts that are quite different than our own.

Hawthorn is said to rule from May 13 to June 9, also known as the fae month and sixth moon of the Celtic year. It is the time of the year that represents the bright dawn, the awakening of nature's abundance and fecundity. It is a twilight time of the year, its opposite being Halloween, another time of twilight or half light. May is a time to connect to the fae energy. Hawthorn is a traditional tree used for maypoles, and its berries are strung together for Beltane festivals (celebrated April 30 to May 1). Hawthorn is one of the nine woods that are traditionally placed on the balefires of Beltane. An old Medieval saying goes: "Hawthorn is burned to purify and draw faerie to your eye . . ."

Hawthorn eases weakness of the stomach and cardiovascular system, and the berries are often prescribed to assist heart health. The tea or tincture of hawthorn leaves and blossoms carries the energy to improve anxiety, appetite loss, poor circulation, and irregular heartbeat; regulate high or low blood pressure; and in some cases, prevent miscarriages. It is a powerful herb used for needs of the heart, including emotional love. Hawthorn seeds can be roasted and used like coffee. The wood from the hawthorn provides the hottest fire known, which is no surprise considering its association with Mars, the Roman God of War. It is used for protection, love and marriage, health and prosperity, fertility, purification, chastity, male potency, purity, inner journeys, intuition, female sexuality, cleansing, and happiness.

Hawthorn flowers can be added to a salad, or even sprinkled on desserts, as the musky scent attracts sensuality for both sexes. The fruits make an excellent wine, again lending its energy to attraction and playfulness.

Sacred hawthorns guard wishing wells in Ireland, where shreds of clothing ("clouties") are hung on the thorns to symbolize a wish made. The Roman goddess Cardea, mistress of Janus, who was keeper of the doors, had as her principal protective emblem a bough of hawthorn. "Her power is to open what is shut; to shut what is open." Hawthorn is also associated with the deities of Flora, the White Goddess Maia, and Hymen.

May Blossom Wine

INGREDIENTS

2 pints (900 grams) hawthorn blossoms,
    stalks trimmed
1 gallon (3.8 liters) boiling water
1 lemon
7 cups (1750 grams) plus 1 teaspoon sugar
1 packet dried all-purpose yeast
1/2 cup (175 milliliters) warm water

Place the blossoms in a bowl and pour over the boiling water. Juice and thinly peel the zest of the lemon and add to the bowl. Cover with a clean cloth and leave for 3 days, stirring twice each day. After 3 days, strain the mixture into a pan, add the 7 cups (1,750 grams) sugar, and bring to a boil. Stir until the sugar is dissolved, and simmer for 10 minutes. Set aside to cool. Put the yeast into a small bowl and add 1/2 cup (125 milliliters) warm water (110 to 130°F or 43 to 54°C) and 1 teaspoon sugar. Allow to cool at room temperature, about 15 minutes or so. Pour the cooled blossom mixture into a fermenting jar, then add the cooled yeast mixture. Be careful not to overfill. Seal the jar and leave in a warm place to ferment for 3 to 6 months.

After 3 to 6 months, strain the mixture and pour the wine into a clean demijohn and cork. When the fermentation is complete, siphon off the residual yeast, and allow to steep for another 6 months to 1 year. Pour into bottles and cork.

Yields approximately four 1-quart (1-liter) bottles

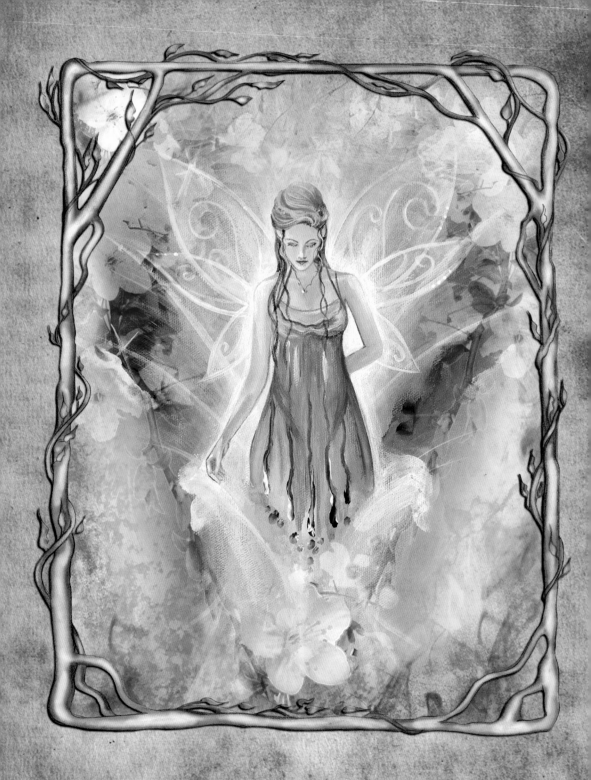

Jasmine

Jasminum (various species)

Jessamin, Moonlight on the Grove

PARTS USED: FLOWERS

There are about 150 species of jasmine as vines or shrubs. The leaves of this plant are most often dark green and mostly ternate, meaning arranged in threes, or pinnate, with the leaves arranged like the veins of a feather. The fragrant flowers are usually white or yellow and tinged with pink. In general, jasmine prefers full to partial sun and frequent watering.

Jasmine increases self-confidence, self-love, spiritual love, compassion, dreams, expansion, and prosperity. It is associated with Diana, Moon Goddess of the Hunt and All Things Wild; Quan Yin, Goddess of Compassion; and Mother Mary. These three female figures all have the ability to nourish and sustain us through whatever difficulties may arise. Quan Yin holds a vessel that contains all the tears ever shed and helps her followers bear their sorrows and pain with the dignity of being supported by a deity witnessing their experience. Ancient Greek worshippers adored Goddess Diana so much that the only way the Christians could rid the people of their goddess was by assimilating her into their new religion. Thus, Ephesus, the home of Diana's Temple, became a place to worship Mary, Mother of God. The amalgam of jasmine's association to the Goddesses of Independence, Compassion, and Nurturing establishes jasmine's faerie essence as the quintessential female energy in its wholeness and perfection.

The fae energy of jasmine calls upon you to draw up the power of Divine Female that once ruled the world. For too long our world has been in imbalance with a focus on outward manifestations and accumulation, and the earth and her creatures are suffering because of it. We must turn inward and find the inner strength of the feminine that lives in all of us, so that from this place of inner knowing we can act from a place of kindness and strength.

Jasmine Body Oil

This oil is recommended for application when you get out of the shower or whenever your soul needs soothing. The carrier oil should be something emollient and thick. Avocado, almond, and jojoba oils are all rich oils, perfect for soothing dry skin. There are two ways to make this oil.

JASMINE

"Within you lies the power of compassion, nurturing, and love. Within me, the essence to help you see this wholeness and perfection, allowing you to be transformed. Come steal away under the beauty of the moon. We shall bloom through the darkness so we may share our delicious fragrance with the world."

INGREDIENTS

8 to 10 drops jasmine essential oil
1 cup (250 milliliters) emollient carrier oil

Drop the essential oil into the carrier oil and shake. This is an easy, modern-goddess recipe that will smell good and carry the vibration of jasmine.

Yields approximately 1 cup (250 milliliters) of infused oil

INGREDIENTS

1 cup (250 milliliters) emollient carrier oil
2 cups (450 grams) dried jasmine flowers

Pack the jasmine flowers into a glass jar. Cover with the carrier oil. Set the jar in the sun for 2 to 4 weeks. Strain the oil into a clean jar.

This process, called an infusion, extracts the plant's most vital life force into the oil, but takes longer. However, you have the chance to work with plants that are closest to their original state, you are naturally going to get the most out of the herb's energy properties in your recipes. You can either dry your own garden jasmine or purchase dried jasmine flowers. Alternately, some dried herbs are available at your local farmers market, herb shop or natural food store.

Yields approximately 1 cup (250 milliliters) of infused oil

Jasmine Scrub

Scrubs are a good way to exfoliate dried skin and stimulate cell renewal, while leaving you feeling silky smooth. Also, while you rub this scrub over your body you can take it a step further and imagine that you are letting go of all resistance to becoming the best of your feminine qualities. Allow the essence of Diana, Quan Yin, and Mother Mary to seep into your pores and become part of who you are.

INGREDIENTS

¼ cup (60 milliliters) jasmine body oil
½ cup (113 grams) organic sugar
¼ teaspoon citric acid
1 teaspoon aloe vera gel
1 teaspoon shea butter

Mix together the jasmine body oil, sugar, citric acid, and aloe vera gel. Gently warm the shea butter. (You can place the shea butter in a shot glass. Then, pour steaming water into a small, shallow dish. Put the shot glass in the dish and within a minute it will melt.) Add the melted butter to the mixture and stir until well mixed. Pour into a clean jar

Yields 1 cup (225 grams)

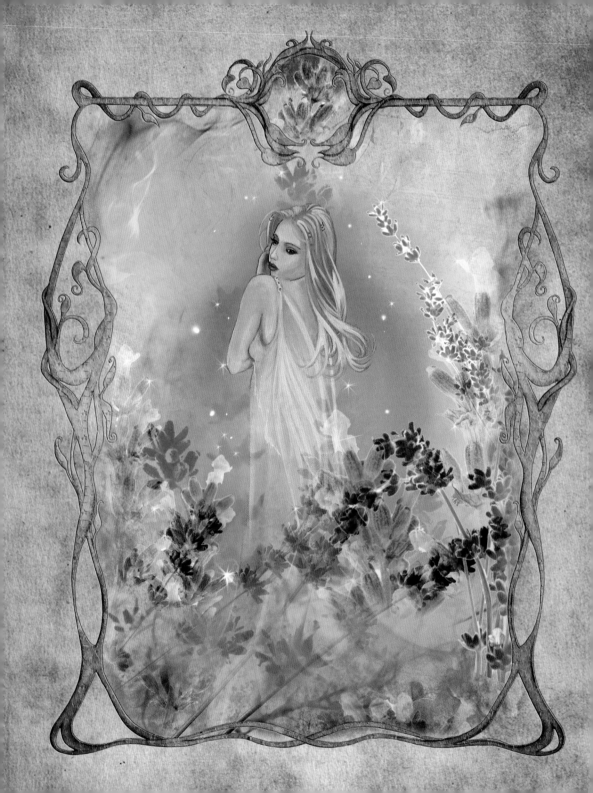

Lavender

Lavandula angustifolia

Elf Leaf, Garden Lavender, Spike, Sticadore, True Lavender

PARTS USED: FLOWERS

There are thirty-nine species of lavender. Lavender has spikes of bluish purple fragrant flowers atop tall thin stems, surrounded by mounds of grayish leaves, and is cultivated primarily in Provence, France. It prefers sandy, coarse soil with good drainage, and a lot of sun.

Lavender is considered to be a powerful herb that attracts energy of a high vibrational nature. It is an antispasmodic, an antidepressant, a nervine relaxant, a muscle relaxant, and an analgesic. Not only is it harvested at midday, when the sun is at its zenith and lavender's oil content is highest, but for centuries it has also been a sacred herb of Midsummer, when the sun's strength is at its most powerful for the entire year. According to ancient lore, it is believed that King Solomon (ruler of Jerusalem from 971–931 BCE) chose lavender to be included in his holy water because of its reputation to cleanse and purify.

The herb is used for meditation, clairvoyance, stability, prosperity, blessing, and calming. Traditionally, lavender was burned in birthing rooms, used to bless homes, woven into wreaths to crown newly married couples, or hung by the bunches throughout the home to dispel flies and mosquitoes.

Today, lavender is widely used in baths, linen closets, perfumes, and soaps for its pure, fresh scent. Lavender is also used as a tea, an infusion, a compress, a flower extract, and an essential oil; in sachets, potpourris, eye pillows, and baths; and as an ingredient in culinary dishes. A couple of sprigs of lavender or lavender flowers in an organza bag tied with raffia embellish a present beautifully and is much more earth-friendly than paper or a plastic bow.

A handful of lavendar in a cloth bag can be used in a bath to relieve tension; or as a compress to relieve cold symptoms, congestion, acne, cysts, and rheumatism and bring relief to insect bites, cuts, wounds, aches, and bruises. A couple of drops of lavender essential oil massaged into the temples will bring cooling relief to migraines or headaches. You can also apply the oil to the bottom of your feet, where the skin is the thinnest and the oil can easily absorb into your bloodstream and correct the imbalance that caused the headache. A lavender steam will alleviate a sinus infection.

Lavender essential oil applied neat (directly on the skin) will relieve first degree burns, irritating skin blemishes, muscle cramps, and insect bites. A couple of drops of oil can be added to your washing machine or dryer to add a fresh scent. Diluted in $^1/_2$ cup (125 milliliters) of water, 10 drops of lavender oil makes an excellent spritz for sunburned skin. For middle ear infections, saturate a cotton ball in olive oil, add 5 drops of lavender oil, and place the cotton ball on the outer part of the affected ear. The lavender oil will help relieve the pain and inhibit the inflammation.

The word *lavender* originates from the Latin *lavare*, which means "to wash." The lavender faerie essence invokes the ability to purify the most holy or darkest of places with precise and irrefutable strength. And yet, lavender accomplishes this feat through such calm and peace that resistance is futile. To further enhance its strength, lavender is associated with the astrological sign of Virgo (independence) and the planets and deities Saturn (father figure and time), Mercury (communication), and Hecate (mystery).

Lavender Chocolate Truffles

The darkness of the chocolate and the freshness of the lavender in these chocolate truffles are a delicious example of tapping into the exquisite power of using purity to slice through shadows, communication to lance mystery, and self-suffiency to thwart limitations.

INGREDIENTS

12 ounces (360 grams) bittersweet chocolate
1 cup (250 milliliters) heavy cream
1 teaspoon dried lavender
1 cup (240 grams) unsweetened cocoa

Grate the chocolate. Bring the cream and the lavender to a simmer in a small saucepan for 1 minute, then strain out the lavender pieces. Add the lavender-cream mixture to the chocolate and stir to melt. Mix well. Chill for at least 3 hours. Roll into 1-inch balls, then roll in cocoa.

Makes 24 truffles

LAVENDER

"I linger along the path of pure bliss. I am peace, here to bring you from chaotic waters or quiet sadness. Let me lead you to the gentle bed of my flowers."

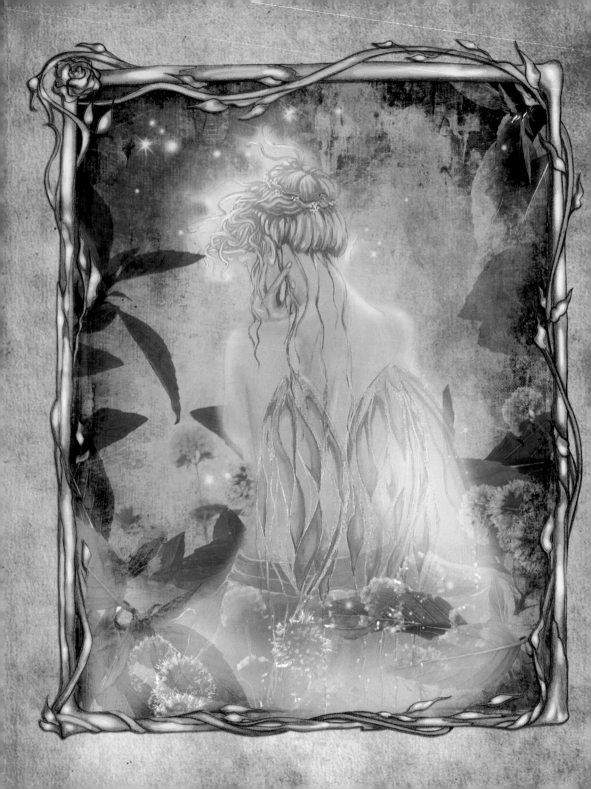

Mint

Mentha (various species)

Brandy Mint, Garden Mint, Lammit, Our Lady's Mint, Yerba Buena

PARTS USED: LEAVES

There are three chief species of mint in cultivation and general use: spearmint (*Mentha viridis*), peppermint (*Mentha piperita*), and pennyroyal (*Mentha pulegium*), the first being the one ordinarily used for cooking. Mint's rough, narrow leaves are very fragrant. It prefers rich, moist, well-drained soil and full sun to partial shade.

Peppermint has the highest number of active agents, including the essential oil menthol, which gives the herb its healing powers. Peppermint can alleviate headaches, migraines, stomach pains, motion sickness, fatigue, stomach cramps, nausea, sore throats, diarrhea, flatulence, or inflamed gums; stimulate liver and gallbladder functions; improve concentration; open nasal passages; and serve as a natural alternative to mouthwash. An infusion of $1/2$ ounce of mint and $1/2$ ounce of red clover with 1 quart (1 liter) of boiling water that is allowed to steep overnight will relieve milk-congested or tender breasts.

As an essential oil, peppermint oil is effective for fighting respiratory infections, but take care to keep your eyes closed when inhaling. You can mix with a carrier oil and massage into the temples and nape of your neck to help relieve a headache or nerve pain. Peppermint oil, when applied to your temples or the bottom of your feet, will provide soothing, relaxing warmth that opens and eases tension. The skin

"In your quiet moments I wish to be with you, soothing and relaxing you, yet revitalizing your spirit. Create that moment where the world washes away and we are present in the now. What a powerful place to be."

is very thin at the bottom of your feet and oils can quickly and easily be absorbed into the bloodstream.

Peppermint tea should never be given to infants or small children and is not recommended for people with heartburn or severe stomach problems due to gastroesophageal reflux disease (GERD). Pregnant and nursing women should avoid using the essential oil.

Lamenting with Minthe

There are times when some form of grief, sadness, anger, guilt, or another emotion takes over. We can try to analyze, dissect, and rationalize it away, but the feeling has immense sticking power and adheres itself to us until we face it once and for all. And yet we avoid traveling to the depths and darkness of our grief because we fear that we will never find our way back out to the light again.

When you give yourself permission to go into the dark, you meet your true self, the observer, the presence without identification through form or personal and familial story. It is in this dark mystery where all the expansiveness and illimitable potential and power of your true and possible self is created. But will you rise from your grief once you begin to wail? Just ask Minthe.

In the Greek myth of Minthe we find what appears to be an evolution of culture, but underneath is an archetypical story of rebirth and rejuvenation through the catharsis of tears. Minthe was a nymph goddess of the River Cocytus, also known as "the river of wailing," which flowed into Hades, the Underworld. The word *cocytus* is a Greek word meaning "lamentation." According to Greek mythos, Minthe had an affair with Hades, the King or God of the Underworld.

When Persephone, Hades's wife, discovered Minthe and Hades were having an affair, she flew into a rage and either she or her mother, Demeter, turned Minthe into dust. From the ashes rose the plant mint. Some legends say that Persephone cursed Minthe and turned her into mint. In this second story, Hades, or Pluto, as he is known in this version, softened the curse by giving mint her aromatic smell, which would intensify when someone brushed against the plant.

The fact that Hades's name changed to Pluto shows that a newer culture took over this story, because Pluto is the Roman name for the God of the Underworld. Ancient Greeks were polyamorous, meaning they had many lovers. Perhaps the Roman culture favored monogamy or wanted to create an original model of a jealous woman—one who could be controlled through her insecurity.

Perhaps Persephone didn't curse Minthe, but blessed her with the ability to live dually, as the guarding energy of the river of tears and wailing, and then transforming her into a plant known for its ability to energize and invigorate. As you enjoy this peppermint tea, imagine yourself as a nymph goddess, able to cry in the darkness, because you know to the core of your being that your sister Persephone, Queen of the Underworld, will help you be reborn as a plant with the energy of being prolific, reviving, and open. This is a calming and restorative tea that will also help settle an upset stomach, which can sometimes precede the tears that need to come.

INGREDIENTS

1/2 cup (113 grams) peppermint leaves
1/2 cup (113 grams) lemon balm leaves
1/2 cup (113 grams) fennel seeds

Use 1 tablespoon of the mixture per cup (250 milliliters) of boiling water. Steep for 10 minutes, then strain.

Yields 1 cup (250 milliliters) of tea

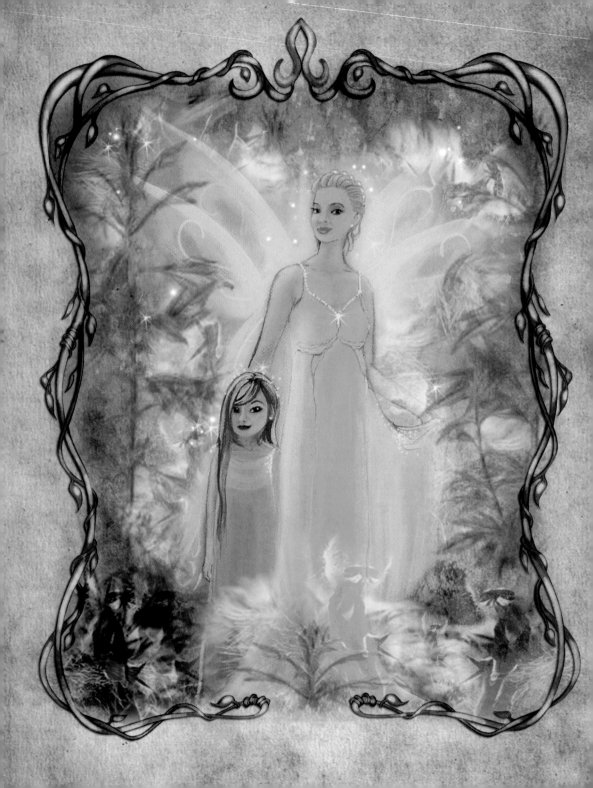

Motherwort

Leonurus cardiaca

Heart Heal, Lionheart, Lion's Ear, Lion's Tail, Mother Herb, Throw-Wort

PARTS USED: FLOWERS, LEAVES, STEMS

Motherwort is a perennial herb with a square stem and lance-shaped leaves. Clusters of small, pink to lilac flowers appear in leaf bases on the upper part of the plant that blooms between June and August. Motherwort can be found along roadsides, banks of rivers and streams, and in vacant fields. It prefers partial shade, but can also grow in full sun and dry soil. In the fall, motherwort produces a large amount of seeds and readily reseeds itself.

For centuries, motherwort gained the reputation for expelling wicked spirits and has been used to dispel doldrums and anxiety. Today, 5 to 10 drops of motherwort tincture will help alleviate mood swings. In China, it has long been taken to lengthen life. Motherwort is used by many herbalists to promote menstrual bleeding and the uterine contractions that lead to childbirth. It is also believed to lower blood pressure. Motherwort not only tones the heart, but also its antispasmodic action relaxes muscles. Its mild sedative effect relieves anxiety, tension, and mood

MOTHERWORT

"My magick happens when you let go of control. I am then free to blow through the world as was intended. Be kind to yourself, for I believe in you. Believe enough to let go."

swings, but does not cause drowsiness. In fact, motherwort effectively treats premenstrual syndrome and menopause. Motherwort must not be used during pregnancy or menstruation, because it can result in heavy bleeding.

If you have sensitive skin, you should avoid handling motherwort.

Motherwort is an excellent herb to help you fortify your trust in others and thereby turn that excess nurturing energy toward yourself. The herb's Latin name, *Leonurus cardiaca*, means "lionhearted." It takes the lion's courage and leadership to teach by example, to allow the ego of savior to die and find the inner strength to be true to yourself, without excess worries over another.

Lionhearted Tea Blend

As you prepare this special tea blend, consider simple things that you can do on a daily basis to nurture your soul and be kind to yourself. For example, you may choose to take a bath, take a walk, read a magazine article, light a candle, listen to music, sun yourself, give yourself a facial, watch the sunset, prepare a favorite meal—heck, sit down to eat. Choose ten things that make you feel content, relaxed, and fulfilled with lighthearted happiness.

Over a week's time, commit to do at least three of these self-nurturing acts every day, including drinking 1 to 2 cups of the tea each day during the week. There is a direct correlation between how well you nurture yourself and how even your temperament is, how physically healthy you are, and how much energy you have.

Recognize where you may have fallen into the tendency to over-mother, to get so far into another's business that you may have lost sight of what is most important in your own life. Perhaps your attention became directed on trying to fix, redirect, or protect another. This behavior, when unbalanced, can cause unnecessary stress due to the fact that we cannot control other people's destiny or prevent them from learning from life's experiences in whatever form is best for them, meaning whatever form will get the message through. The Great Cosmic two-by-four smacked against the forehead hurts. But sometimes, the best way for some people to learn is from life's hard knocks rather than the gentle nudges. And our concerns and efforts to save them from themselves, however kindhearted, can, in fact, be downright demoralizing.

When our nurturing becomes invasive, we send the message that we do not trust that the other person can function or handle life without our intervention. When we constantly shield or minimize life's difficulties for another, we can have the effect of kryptonite—weakening the life force of another by our intense distrust of her own inherent strength. We can do this to spouses, younger siblings, friends, and children. Even young children need to be taught age-appropriate tasks of self-care to develop a healthy self-esteem.

This ritual is about you letting go of your need to be that Great Cosmic Mother for another and trust that the Divine Feminine is big enough and strong enough to take care of all. Imagine that you are letting go of all the people, situations, and events. Visually see yourself opening your hands and dropping everything that does not make you feel energized when you think of it. As you release, imagine a wind that picks up and carries the responsibilities to the Great Mother. She has them now. She will take care of them with the strength and wisdom of the Goddess. And she supports you to be the woman you have longed to be.

INGREDIENTS
1/4 cup (55 grams) dried motherwort leaves
1/4 cup (55 grams) hawthorn berries
1/4 cup (55 grams) dried lemon balm leaves

Pour 1 cup (250 milliliters) of boiling water over 1 teaspoon of the lionhearted tea blend, steep for 10 minutes, and strain.

Yields 1 cup (250 milliliters) of tea

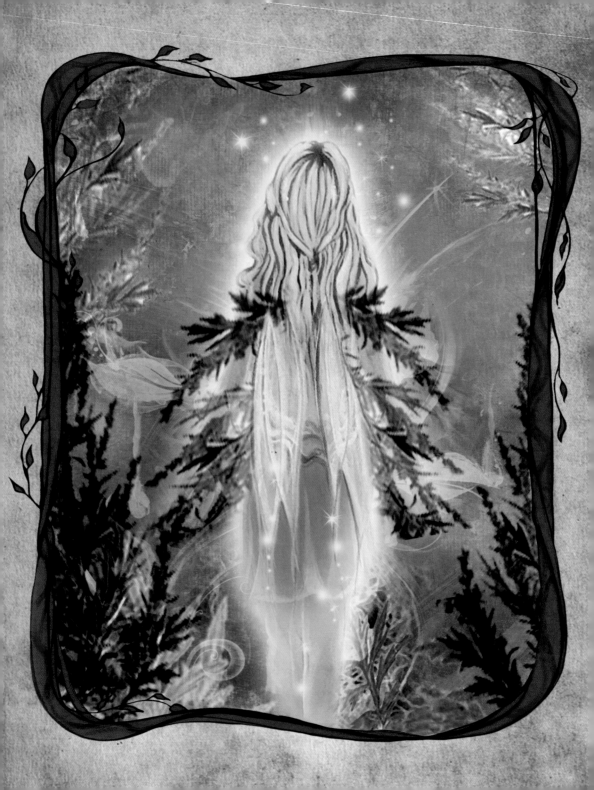

Mugwort

Artemisia vulgaris

Artemis Herb, Chrysanthemum Weed, Felon Herb, Old Uncle Harry,
Sailor's Tobacco, St. John's Plant, Wild Wormwood, Witch Herb

PARTS USED: LEAVES, ROOTS

Mugwort is a perennial shrub with angular stems, often of a purplish hue, that grow 3 feet or more in height. The pointed leaves are smooth and of a dark green tint on the upper surface, but covered with a dense, silver cottony down beneath. The flowers are in small oval heads and are either reddish or pale yellow. Some believe that mugwort received its name from once being a major flavoring in beverages, a.k.a., "mug herb." Mugwort prefers full sun and average to poor soil. It is best to gather mugwort during a full moon in late summer.

Mugwort is well known for being an emmenagogue, meaning it aids the menstrual cycles, whether it is needed to regulate or stimulate menses flow, relieve cramps, prevent or terminate early pregnancy, promote easy labor, or restore health after childbirth. This herb is also used as a nervine, a diaphoretic, an aromatic, a diuretic, and a stimulant. It helps heal minor skin abrasions. Simply chew a mugwort leaf and a plantain leaf and place over the scrape and cover with a bandage or clear tape. The chewing releases the herb's healing, volatile oils and one's own saliva speeds the process of recovery.

For centuries, mugwort has been used as a tool to aid prophecy and divination, protection, particularly during travel, and consecrating or blessing. It is strongly connected to the crystal ball. It has been used in dream pillows to induce happy, prophetic dreams. In China, during the Dragon Festival on the fifth day of the fifth moon, mugwort was hung on a person to protect him from evil spirits. During the Middle Ages it was worn also for protection, particularly on St. John's Eve.

By virtue of its Latin name, *Artemisia vulgaris*, mugwort is strongly associated with Artemis, the maiden goddess, associated with the woods, the wild, the moon, cunning, independence, and freedom, and primarily a protectress of girls. Artemis is eternally young, lithe, and proud—a tomboy who never grows up. She carries a bow with her and her skill is unsurpassed. She is a supreme athlete with a concentrated will, who has been called upon by Olympians far and wide for three thousand consecutive years.

Artemis's connection with the moon unites her with dreams and prophecy; however, she is also associated with logic, precision, and action. It is interesting that the underside of mugwort is silver like the moon and the plant helps women in a very specific way. Many women in ancient Greece prayed to Artemis as the celestial midwife, who was said to often appear at the childbed in visionary form, carrying a flaming pine torch as symbolic of protective warmth.

MUGWORT

"Some say you can't see the forest through the trees. I can. Let's jump into your dreams and see what we can conjure!"

Artemis-Mugwort Vision for New Birth

During a new moon or when the sliver of the moon has just appeared, set aside time for a special visualization with Artemis and mugwort. Prepare yourself by fasting for at least 3 hours prior to this meditation. After the moon has risen or when it is completely dark, sit outside where you feel protected. If possible, light four candles and place them in the four cardinal directions to act as protectors for you as you slip into the meditative state. Be certain to use tealight candles, advent candles, or candles that cannot blow over and cause a fire.

In a bowl, sprinkle 3 tablespoons of mugwort leaves and 3 tablespoons of pine leaves into fresh springwater. You can also use essential oil or either or both herbs. Take three deep calming breaths. Allow the thoughts to come in and flow out. Now begin to focus on the third eye, or point on the forehead between your eyes. Say:

"Artemis, Goddess of Will and the Hunt,
Grant me the strength to focus on my dream.
Give me the courage to stand with you,
Whether in woods, meadow, or stream."

Visualize a silvery green luminescence before you. Smell the pine scent in the air, reminiscent of Artemis's many hunts through the forest. She is wild and free, and without complications she can bring your desire to you. Watch as a green light shimmers off her and enters your auric field through your heart center. Now visualize the dream you would have manifest. Imagine that the new thing that you want— a lover, a new job, a new home, a baby, financial security, or a creative endeavor. Ask Artemis's help in attaining your dream. Imagine that she is your midwife in the birth of your greatest desire. Welcome all the feelings of wellness this new birth will bring you. When you feel complete in this visualization, imagine a flaming pine torch appears in Artemis's hand, and she gives it to you. Hear her say:

"All that you wish is granted,
By my will, so may it be."

Sit with Artemis as long as you like. Call in her strength as your strength. Know that her will and confidence are with you. Think about all the good you can do with your met desire. Realize that her precision is yours, for when you call upon the strength of Artemis and mugwort, nothing can stand in your way.

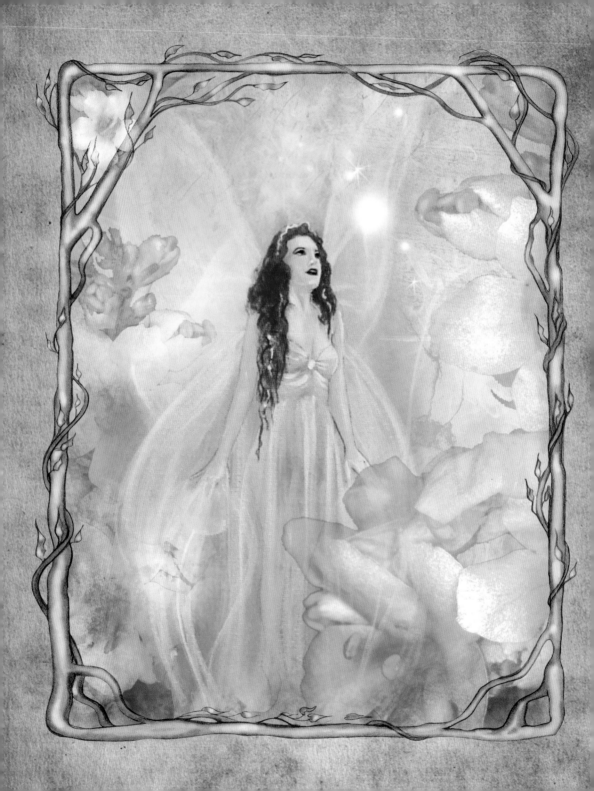

Mullein

Verbascum (various species)

Aaron's Rod, Adam's Flannel, Beggar's Stalk, Blanket Leaf,
Bullock's Lungwort, Candlewick Plant, Cuddy's Lungs, Duffle,
Fettwort, Fluffweed, Golden Rod, Hag's Taper, Hare's Beard,
Jacob's Staff, Jupiter's Staff, Lady's Foxglove, Old Man's Flannel,
Peter's Staff, Ray Paper, Torches, Velvet Dock, Wild Ice Leaf, Woolen

PARTS USED: LEAVES, FLOWERS

Mullein is known for its broad, downy, grayish leaves. After its second year, yellow, rose-like flowers grow on tall spikes and have a honey scent. Mullein prefers well-drained loam, little to moderate watering, and full sun. It can reach up to 6 feet, especially in very sunny locations. New plants can be propagated by seed or root cuttings in late winter. Most mullein varieties will self-seed freely. The herb's Latin name, *verbascum*, is most likely derived from the Latin word *barba*, meaning "beard," which very well relates to mullein's shaggy appearance.

Mullein is used as an antiseptic, analgesic, and expectorant in the form of a tea, an infusion, an extract, and a tincture. It has a soothing quality that affects the digestive tract, mucous membranes, and the lymphatic system. Mullein has been used to treat internal ailments such as chronic colds, bronchitis, coughs, pneumonia, tuberculosis, bowel disorders, headaches, sinus troubles, cystitis, laryngitis, tonsillitis, and asthma. It can alleviate external problems such as bedsores, joint pain, sores in the mouth and throat, burns, and hemorrhoids. The plant has also been used to aid poor sleeping. It is often combined with garlic in tinctures to aid earaches.

Due to the fact that it grows very tall spikes, sometimes well overhead, traditionally mullein stalks have been dipped in tallow and used as a torch in outdoor festivities. This custom is particularly popular during All Hallow's Eve. Today, the tall spikes are not lit, but are used to symbolize fire and the southern direction. This particular usage explains some of the plant's interesting folk names, such as candlewick plant, hag's taper, and torches. In addition, the plant's leaves feel like coarse velvet, another attribute contributing to its nicknames, like blanket leaf, velvet dock, and woolen. Some monasteries grew mullein as a means of protection against evil. The powdered leaves are known as "graveyard dust" and are used in ancient magickal recipes. The herb is often planted alongside homes to ward off lightning. Although mullein is associated with the planet and god Saturn, typically an earth-centered deity, this plant is also related to the energy of fire.

Speaking Your Truth

Mullein is most often used to heal chronic coughs, dry coughs, and hoarseness. Excessive coughing is a result of an obstruction of the throat chakra—the energy center that controls our ability to express ourselves. Coughing is a way to get attention, to bark out the things we most want to say, but for some reason, the words get caught in our throat. Mullein will help you move through the obstruction with the determination of Saturn and the will of fire.

This ritual will help you open your throat chakra and speak those difficult words in a way that communicates precisely what your heart most wants to say. Once you break through the emotional walls and the scarring in your throat, you will find coughs begin to fade and a healing occurs. On a Saturday, the day of the week dedicated to Saturn, find a quiet place to sit and meditate. Imagine a cooling, soothing color filling the space around and within your throat. Begin to hum. Get accustomed to the sound of your voice, however large or small it is. Simply accept your sound.

Now drop 2 full droppers of mullein tincture in $^{1}/_{2}$ cup (125 milliliters) water. You may also choose to make an infusion of mullein (1 cup or 225 grams fresh herb, covered with water and allowed to sit for 4 hours or overnight, then drained). Drink the water or infusion and feel the milky smoothness coat your throat. As the soothing sensation fills the back of your throat and trickles down, imagine your throat opening and expanding. Feel all the restrictions fall away as you continue to open.

MULLEIN

"Sing songs of truth from love and I will join you. The magick in our voices will ring through the air and bring us joy and peace. Let me guide you through the flames of unspoken need to the soothing waters of release."

After a few sips, visualize a fire representing courage glowing in your belly. Begin to hum again. Notice whether there are any changes to your throat. Chant "Om" three times, followed by a repetition of the words "I am that I am" three times. Finish your mullein water. Without using specific words (unless they pop into your mind effortlessly), imagine that the intention of what you need to tell someone is communicated seamlessly and successfully. Your open communication has created understanding, respect, and a win-win for everyone. You do not need to imagine the exact words you need to say to another person to experience the peace in this ritual. This ceremony is designed to give you the experience of an opening, soothing sensation to the throat chakra, which will naturally allow this energy center to do what it does best—communicate from love. The medicine of this plant will work on you without you needing to direct the energy. You will find that your words are precise and true, in line with the will of Saturn.

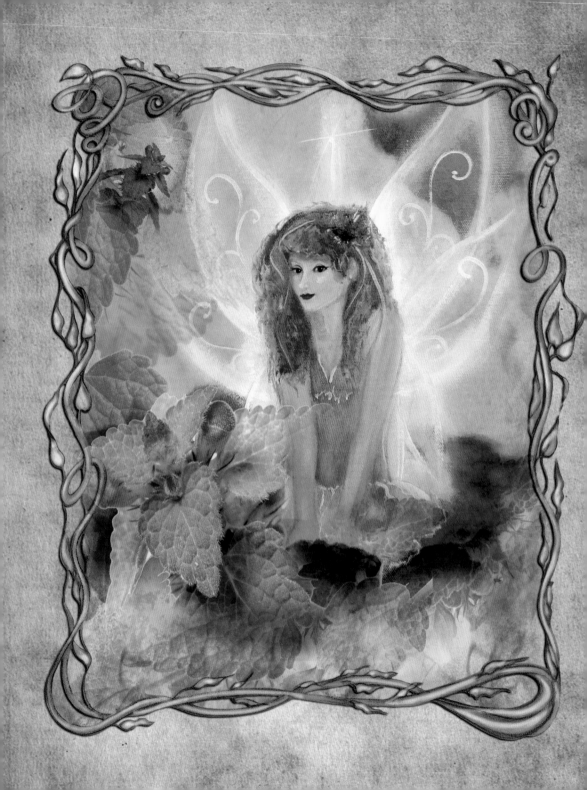

Nettle

Urtica dioica

Stinging Nettle, Wild Spinach

PARTS USED: LEAVES, ROOTS, SEEDS, FLOWERS, STALKS

nettle leaves are serrated, hairy, and dull green and have formic acid that burns the skin. Nettle prefers rich, moist soil and full sun to partial shade.

Interestingly, the irritating toxin found in nettle leaves that chafes the skin is responsible for its renowned healing effects. Nettle is well known for its tonic effect on the nervous system. It has also traditionally been used for protection. Its faerie energy calms and soothes while it protects.

Nettle has been used to treat colds, gout, and stomachaches. It can stem bleeding, including nosebleeds, heavy menstrual flow, and wounds. Nettle has been used as a gargle to soothe sore throats. Nettle tea (3 to 4 teaspoons dried nettle leaves to 1 cup [250 milliliters] hot water, then steeped for 10 minutes) alleviates diarrhea, dysentery, kidney stones, arthritis, and hemorrhoids; prevents premature hair loss; and helps lower blood sugar levels. This tea is effective in treating a cold before it matures, stemming illness in the stage of chills, runny nose, and general discomfort. It can quench thirst and, due to its detoxifying properties, produce a fresh and clear complexion.

A nettle infusion, which consists of 1 ounce herb (or roughly a handful) and 1 quart (1 liter) water that has steeped for 2 hours or overnight, has a somewhat creamy taste and feels soft on the throat as well as the stomach. An excellent source of iron, this chlorophyll-rich plant has high levels of calcium, silica, as well as other minerals and vitamins. This infusion strengthens the adrenals, eases anxiety, increases energy, alleviates the lethargy associated with anemia, helps prevent night sweats, builds blood, protects the heart, and helps with water retention. According to lore, bathing one's hand in a nettle infusion will attract fish. California Native Americans fed their babies nettle tea in the belief it would make them immune to the sting of the plant's leaves.

NETTLE

"To play with me can be dangerous, as I can surely sting you. But remember this: the risk of the sting is worth the healing in the end. Are you willing to step into risk with me?"

Do not use a nettle tea cure for longer than 4 weeks. It should not be used by those with a weakened heart.

Human hair is considered a source of power in many cultures, both in the past and in the present. In particular, it is the power that flows from the crown chakra, also known as the seventh chakra. The chakras are energy centers located throughout the body. There are seven chakras that line up along the spine. The first chakra is located at the perineum floor and relates to security. The second chakra is located at the sexual organs and relates to creativity and individuality. The third chakra is located at the solar plexus and relates to willpower. The fourth chakra is located at the heart center and relates to unconditional love. The fifth chakra is located at the throat and relates to speaking your truth. The sixth chakra is located at the brow and relates to seeing with a unified focus. The seventh chakra, at the top of your head, connects you to higher levels of spirituality.

Nettle is also connected to the god and planet Mars, who rules over action and is often associated with war, although this wasn't always the case. In Roman times, Mars was called Marspiter (Father Mars); however, in his original state, Mars was known as Mars Gradivus (from *grandiri*, meaning "to grow"). Mars was the son of Juno, the Roman mother-goddess, who created a union not with a man but with a flower, to produce Mars. The strength of this infusion will multiply when you consider the herb's lore. Draw upon nettle's history and its associations as you begin to visualize the energy of growth, harmony of all living things, protection, and right action in your life.

Nettle Hair Tonic

While you are preparing this hair tonic and later when you drink it, light a green candle to represent growth and the fae's protection. Shake the jar and say:

> *"I grow slowly as the wild plants grow,*
> *Feeling at peace with life's ebb and flow.*
> *I experience joy as my divine right,*
> *And bathe in love's protection and light."*

INGREDIENTS

4 drops nettle essential oil or ¹/₂ cup (113 grams) dried nettle leaves
4 drops lavender essential oil or ¹/₄ cup (55 grams) fresh lavender flowers
4 drops rosemary essential oil or ¹/₄ cup (55 grams) fresh rosemary leaves
  (for dark hair, substitute with calendula, and use chamomile for light hair)
4 drops cedarwood essential oil
1 cup (250 milliliters) coconut oil, slightly warmed, so it liquefies

Mix the oils together. (If you are using plant matter, pour the oil over the herbs and allow to sit for 1 week, then drain and save the oil. You can also use a combination of fresh herbs and oils, depending on what you have on hand.) Apply directly to your scalp and rub in a clockwise direction. Bring the oil all the way down to the ends of your hair and imagine that wisdom and knowledge are working their way through your entire being, through your emotional, physical, and mental bodies. Braid your hair if it's long enough. Keep the oil in as long as you can, overnight if possible. You may want to put a bath towel over your pillow to protect your pillowcase. Oiling your hair prevents split ends and after washing it, leaves your hair luxurious and silky smooth.

Yields 1 cup (250 milliliters) of hair tonic

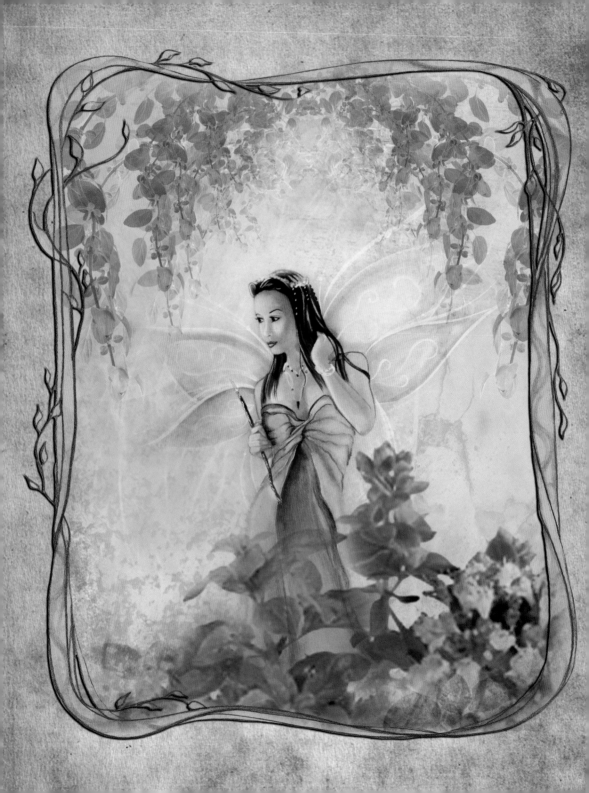

Oregano

Origanum vulgare

Organy, Origano, Sweet Marjoram

PARTS USED: LEAVES

Oregano is a low-lying perennial herb with hairy, erect, square stems; oval, pointed leaves; and two-lipped flowers that range in color from white to purple. Oregano likes full sun and ordinary, well-drained soil.

Oregano is used widely in the culinary dishes of Greece, Spain, Italy, Portugal, the Caribbean, and Mexico. The name *oregano* is derived from the Greek words *oro ganos*, which means "joy of the mountains." Coupled with its association with the god and planet Mars, oregano carries the faerie essence of pleasurable action. It brings a delightful, uplifting feeling to most situations. Traditional folk uses include mixing dried oregano leaves with honey to help fade bruises, and chewing leaves to alleviate minor toothaches. It has been used to keep milk sweet, hence its nickname sweet marjoram. It is said that oregano became popular in America when returning World War II soldiers brought back with them a hankering for the "pizza herb."

Oregano has been used to treat coughs, insect bites, tired muscles, asthma, rheumatism, and irregular menstruation. It is also prescribed to aid indigestion, flatulence, bloating, and stomach pains.

As an essential oil, oregano is one of the most powerful and versatile oils. It contains strong immune-enhancing and antioxidant properties and supports the respiratory system. Oregano is a key oil used in the Raindrop Technique, a massage application of powerful antibacterial, antiviral essential oils dropped along the spine. This technique, based on Lakota Native healing, was designed to bring about electrical alignment of the body.

Oregano oil is a natural way to clear viruses and bacteria. Often muscular pain and discomfort can actually be caused by a dormant virus trapped in the muscular tissue. Oregano oil, diluted with a base oil and applied directly to a sore or tense area during a massage, can help clear and eliminate the virus, leaving the recipient pain-free and with more mobility. The oil is increasingly being used to alleviate sinus congestion. Simply apply a few drops of the essential oil with a teaspoon of olive oil to the occipital bulb at the back of your neck and the muscles along the skull at the hairline to help relieve the tension.

The herb has a long history in folk medicine for promoting the onset of menses and should be avoided by pregnant women.

Oregano Love Bread

Oregano enhances meats, eggs, and cheese dishes like quiches, omelets, and frittatas. A simple recipe of one or two bunches of chopped oregano, one or two cloves of crushed garlic and two sticks of sweet butter blended together will complement soups, salads, and pasta dishes. Oregano combines well with garlic, thyme, parsley, and olive oil. A sprig or two of oregano in your morning eggs will add a delicious Mediterranean taste.

Oregano is thought to be precious to the Greek goddess Aphrodite, Goddess of Love. It was said to comfort the dead when it grew on their graves. If you anoint yourself with oregano before sleeping, you will dream of your future spouse. Make this bread with the intention of sharing your love with another and ignite the fae energy of pleasurable action.

INGREDIENTS

½ cup (113 grams) shelled sunflower seeds

¾ cup (170 grams) grated Romano cheese

2 tablespoons chopped oregano leaves

6 cups (720 grams) all-purpose or
  bread flour

1 package rapid-rise dry yeast

1 tablespoon salt

2 tablespoons sugar

2 tablespoons vegetable oil

2 cups (500 milliliters) warm water

1 handful cornmeal

OREGANO

"You caught me with my wand today! With this I can bring much pleasure to you, from your palate to your love interest. Which do you prefer? Maybe both? Oh, the fun we are going to have!"

With a mortar and pestle, grind the sunflower seeds. Mix the ground seeds, cheese, and oregano into the flour. In a large bowl, combine the yeast, flour, salt, sugar, and oil. Add the water, and mix well. Turn out the dough onto a floured surface. Knead for 10 to 15 minutes. Place in a lightly oiled bowl, turn over a couple of times, cover with a warm cloth, and let rise for 10 to 15 minutes.

Preheat the oven to 350°F (177°C). Cover a cookie sheet with the cornmeal. Turn the dough out onto a floured surface, and pat down into a circle. Flatten to at least 1-inch (2.5 centimeters) thickness, and 10 to 12 inches (25 to 30 centimeters) in diameter. Mold the dough into a heart shape. Transfer to the cookie sheet. Bake for 25 to 35 minutes, or until golden brown.

Serves 8

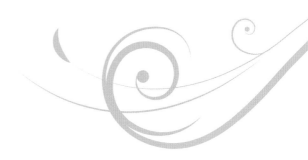

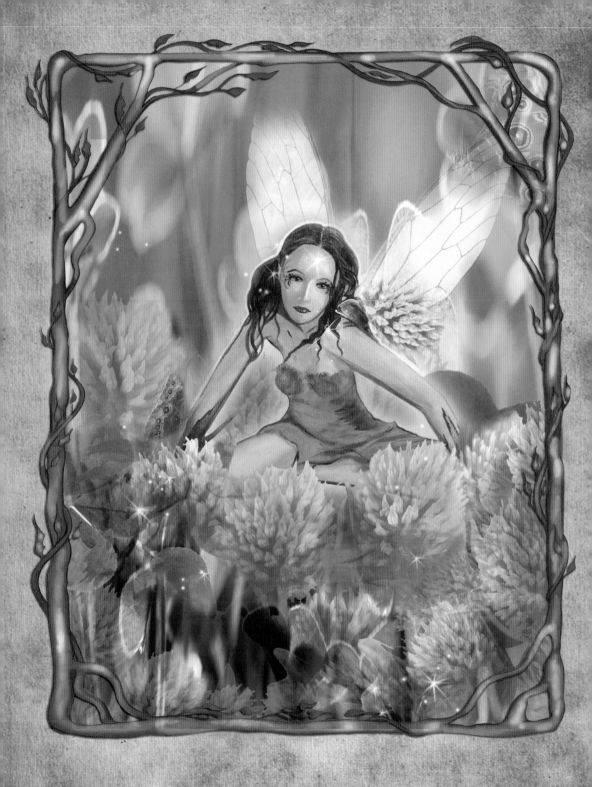

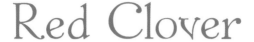

Red Clover

Trifolium pratense

Bee Bread, Cow Clover, Honeystalks, Prize Herb,
Three-Leaves Grass, Trefoil

PARTS USED: FLOWERS, LEAVES

Red clover has hairy stems that grow both erect and sprawling. The leaves are alternate and trifoliate, meaning they have three leaflets together. The characteristic rose pink flower is shaped rather like a puffball. Red clover requires deep water until established and prefers full to partial sun. It is a helpful plant in the garden because it restores nitrogen to the soil.

Red clover is a favorite herb among herbalists, in particular because it cleanses the blood and thereby promotes good circulation. Blood is the essential life force that brings nutrients and oxygen to our entire system. It helps move healthy, germ-fighting cells to disease in the body and flushes the body of toxins. It is a sacred herb among the ancient Celts and was believed to be an Herb of Immortality. Red clover's signature three-leaf foliage has been connected to the Triple Goddess of Maiden, Mother, and Crone as well as the Christian symbol of the trinity. The fae essence of red clover is found in its symbols of life's constant evolution and rebirth.

Red clover is used to treat colds and coughs, soothe nerves, restore vitality, and induce sleep. Topically, red clover has proven to be an effective treatment for eczema and psoriasis and, as a compress, it can speed the healing of minor wounds and relieve insect bites and stings. Red clover has been used to treat anemia with dizziness and palpitations; menstrual disorders, amenorrhea, and dysmenorrhea; constipation; rheumatic arthralgia; traumatic injuries; and carbuncles, boils, and sores. Red clover tea or infusion stimulates the appetite and brings a reprieve from coughs. It is also used to treat various forms of cancer.

It is used magickally for banishing, protection, clear sight, and love. It brings calm and works as a tonic for the body and soul.

In the seventeenth century, the juice of red clover was valued as a cure for eye diseases. The oval-shaped leaflets, with their white spot in the center, resembled the human eye, and a commonly held belief of the time was the Doctrine of Signatures, which stated that if a plant looked like a body part, it was certain to be a cure for it. The leaves and blossoms were also boiled with lard and used as an ointment for cuts, bites, and venomous stings. Perhaps lesser known is the fact that red clover is also an effective agent for eczema, psoriasis, and acne.

RED CLOVER

"We are of this earth, you and I. Our bodies belong to the earth. We are of the same energetic field, for we are all a part of a greater consciousness. Knowing this, let us work together as partners to bring the feminine essence to the surface."

Winter Wonder Cream

Red clover is included in this nighttime cream to reduce the possibility of an acne breakout and is especially effective for use during the colder months, when winter weather actually dries our skin, sometimes making it flaky. This velvety smooth cream also contains calendula, which will address abrasions due to scratching itchy, dry skin. The rose will help maintain the skin's elasticity.

This cream is primarily for nighttime use. Apply immediately after washing your face, or taking a shower, which will trap the water and increase moisture in your skin.

INGREDIENTS

1/3 cup (80 milliliters) red clover-infused oil*
1/3 cup (80 milliliters) calendula-infused oil*
1/3 cup (80 milliliters) rose hip seed oil
3 tablespoons beeswax
1 tablespoon cocoa butter
1/3 cup (80 milliliters) rose geranium hydrosol
1 tablespoon vegetable glycerin
1 teaspoon vitamin E oil
20 drops lavender essential oil

In a small saucepan or double boiler over low heat, warm the base oils, beeswax, and cocoa butter until the wax and butter are just melted. In a separate pan, warm the hydrosol and glycerin. Remove both pans from the heat and allow them to cool to body temperature, until the oil/wax mixture just begins to thicken but is still liquid.

Quickly drizzle the hydrosol and glycerin into the oil/wax mixture while whisking rapidly for 2 to 4 minutes, until a pale yellow emulsion forms. Add the vitamin E oil and essential oil, and rapidly whisk for another 4 to 5 minutes, until the mixture cools and becomes creamy. (I don't use a blender, because this gives my forearms a good workout!)

Spoon the cream into glass jars. Allow the cream to set for about an hour prior to use. This cream's rejuvenating properties are highly concentrated, so you'll only need a pea-sized amount to cover the face and throat.

Yields approximately 1 cup (240 grams)

Both of the herb-infused oils are created by filling a quart-size (1-liter) jar with dried herbs and covering with a base oil, such as jojoba, almond, or avocado. Allow the herb oil to infuse for at least 2 weeks—the longer, the better. You can simply then dip a tablespoon into the jar to collect the oil. Some of the petals will get in the oil, but that's okay.

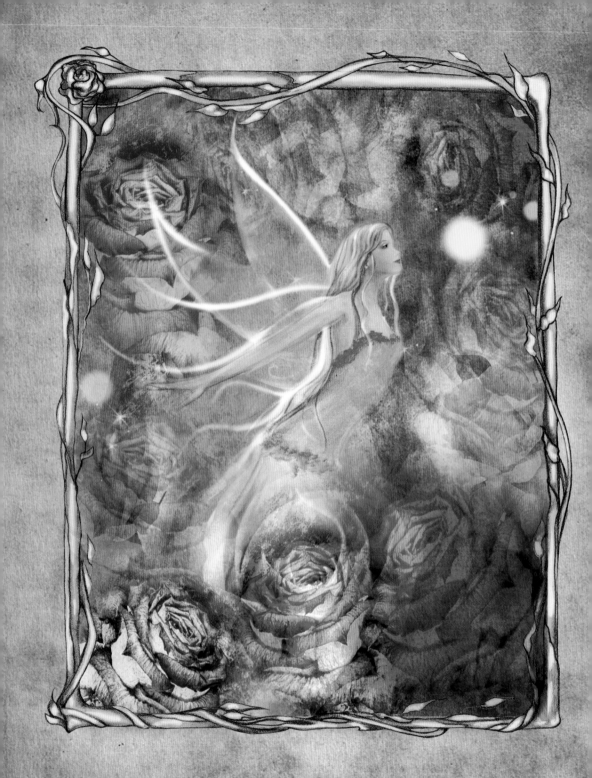

Rose

Rosa (various species)

Field Rose, Hundred-Leaved Rose, Queen of the Garden, Red Rose

PARTS USED: FLOWERS, HIPS

Rose is considered to be one of the few perfect plants, meaning it has roots, leaves, stems, blossoms, and fruit. Roses prefer clay-based, well-drained soil and full sun to partial shade, depending on the species and growing region. They thrive when fed well and often. Ashes from your fireplace or even gray water (reusable water from rinsing dishes) can benefit roses.

The faerie essence of rose has a commanding yet gentle presence. It can bring healing to a volatile or painful arena with its alluring, peaceful scent that infuses us with the knowledge that all will be well. The oil promotes overall emotional and physical healing, heals wounds, promotes well-being, lifts depression, arouses passion, cleanses the skin, and calms the nerves. It has anti-inflammatory, germicidal, and antispasmodic properties.

Rose hips, particularly of the dog rose and other types of wild and shrub roses, emerge in the fall, after the blooms have faded and the petals have dropped off. The hips have a slightly sour but pleasant taste and are prized for their

ROSE

"I am thrilled to finally share myself with you, to show you there is more to me than just my petals and fragrance. Thank you for looking beyond the beauty and even the thorns, to see the substance of me. Such a gift it is surely to be seen."

vitamin C content, which is actually higher than that of citrus fruits. Rose hips also have vitamin A, E, and K, as well as pectin and organic acids. Rose hips are used to treat mild urinary-tract irritation, flu, water retention, rheumatism, and abdominal cramping.

Rose is an excellent herb to work with to invoke love, patience, and trust. When we sit in the mystery, awaiting for life to unfold, there are times we want to rush forward at top speed looking for answers. There can be discomfort sitting in the unknown. But the true potentiality of life exists in these moments of mystery, when anything is possible. We didn't come here to earth to rest on our laurels in sedation with perfect foresight. We came to create out of the mystery and field of possibility.

We often forget that life is a pattern of birth, death, and rebirth. The wisdom of the rose illustrates the need to sit for a time in the dark and stillness of Mother Earth. Then, ever so slowly, the rose moves from a tight bud into full blossom. The petals fall away and become compost for the process to begin again. As we constantly birth a new self, it is best to avoid pushing too hard, too fast—you just might tear, and that's never good, plus it really, really hurts. It's much wiser to follow nature's example and allow yourself to open gradually, trusting in the mystery.

Rose Cordial

INGREDIENTS

6 quarts (6 liters) pure filtered water
I cup (225 grams) chopped, dried rosehips
3 cups (675 grams) dried elderberries
³/₄ cup (170 grams) dried hawthorn berries
¹/₂ cup (113 grams) roselle calyxes (*Hibiscus sabdariffa*)
2 tablespoons dried rhodiola root
I¹/₂ to 2 cups (375 to 500 milliliters) unfiltered wildflower honey, to taste

Combine all the ingredients, except for the honey, and bring to a boil. Cover, lower heat, and simmer for 1 hour. Let the pot sit, covered, overnight. In the morning, reheat, then allow the contents to cool just enough to strain out the berries, but still warm enough to dissolve the honey. Ladle out 2 cups (500 milliliters) of the cordial and strain through a fine-meshed strainer into a 1-quart (1-liter), heat-resistant glass measuring cup. Dissolve the honey into the warm, strained cordial, then return the sweetened cordial back to the pot. Stir until the sweetened, strained cordial and the unsweetened, unstrained cordial are thoroughly incorporated.

In batches, ladle the cordial mixture through a mesh strainer back into the heat-resistant measuring cup, dispose of the botanicals remaining in the strainer, and add them to your compost pile. Pour the freshly strained cordial into clean glass bottles, cap, and refrigerate. Repeat this process until all the cordial is bottled.

Yields about seven 24-ounce (750-milliliter) bottles

When chilled, this cordial is lovely by itself or with a little sparkling mineral water added to it. This recipe can be simplified by omitting the hawthorn berries and rhodiola root. It is nonalcoholic, though it would ferment beautifully.

Although this cordial is healthful and delicious, it should never be given to infants under one year of age, as it contains honey, which in rare instances can contribute to a type of infant botulism.

Notes on the ingredients: Hawthorn berries tone the heart muscle. Rose hips and hibiscus are both high in pectin and vitamin C. Hibiscus is used for its fiber and as a dye, as well as to flavor rose hip teas. Both elderberries and hibiscus are high in antho-cyanins and bioflavonoids, which are very good for our vascular health as well as our eyesight. Elderberries (and hibiscus flowers) are occasionally used as natural dyes, so be careful not to spill this cordial on clothing; the stains will not come out. Elderber-ries have antiviral properties. Wild honey is good to help prevent allergies, and it has antibacterial properties, too. Rhodiola root is an adaptogen often used by Russian athletes to enhance sports performance and prevent stress-related physical disorders. *The beverage was developed by Sabine, Earth Mama, to restore low energy levels.*

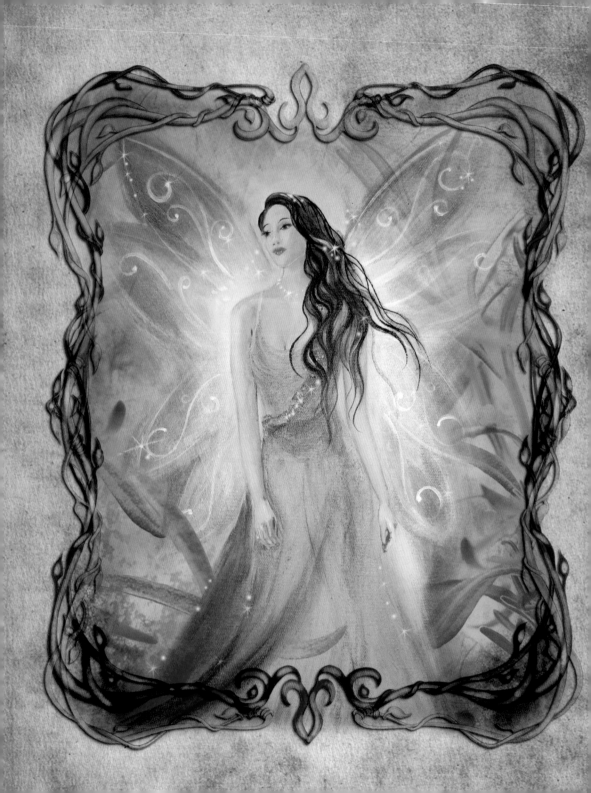

Rosemary

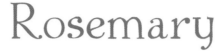

Rosmarinus officinalis

Compass Plant, Dew of the Sea, Guardrobe,
Incensier, Polar Plant, Rosmarie, Sew Dew

PARTS USED: LEAVES, FLOWERS

Rosemary leaves are dark green, small, hard, shiny, and quite aromatic. Its flowers are lipped, small, and vary in color from silvery to dark blue. Rosemary grows well under the full sun and dew. It prefers loose, permeable, well-drained soil. The flowers attract many bees (symbols of fertility and community).

Rosemary derives its name from the Latin word *marinus*, meaning "near the sea." Its association with water establishes rosemary's faerie essence as formidable, yet adaptable and flexible. Like water, the rosemary plant has a malleable quality—it can be shaped into a square or circle or topiary, though this requires diligence because the rosemary grows woody stems in all directions, revealing the need for movement to maintain vitality and avoid stagnation. It is said that rosemary will grow particularly well in gardens tended by strong-willed women.

Rosemary has been used for purification, love, protection, abundance, weather, grounding, and intellect. It has dispelled depression, healed migraines and sore throats, relieved rheumatism and anxiety, been used as a heart tonic, and aided pregnant and lactating mothers. Young brides traditionally carried a sprig of rosemary in their wreaths or wedding bouquets. For centuries, the fragrant herb has been exchanged between friends as a symbol of loyalty and tossed onto the graves of departed loved ones. Gypsy travelers used rosemary as a rinse for highlighting dark hair or as a rejuvenating face wash. It was burned in sickrooms as a disinfectant and was used to ward off the plague.

Of all its uses, rosemary is often best known for its ability to stimulate memory. To remember is to piece together yourself, to bring yourself into wholeness. To remember all that you are is to recall your connection to All That Is—never as a separate being or a part of, but the entirety of the universe, living as you, a unique and important expression of divinity.

Rosemary also restores energy and revitalizes the soul as well as tired bodies. When you are stressed out or feeling depleted and need to remember all that you are, the rosemary fae invite you to spend time in nature, whatever time you can allow for a walk or to just relax. Take a sprig of rosemary with you or bring along rosemary oil. Allow your mind to quiet. Smell your rosemary sprig or oil, breathing in the healing balm of nature. Know that you have the ability to adapt and yet the strength of water to withstand pressure. Keep the oil and sprig with you as you return to your daily routine. Whenever you need to recall your strength or flexibility or just the presence of nature, smell the rosemary and the fae energy will carry you back to a place of well-being.

Those with high blood pressure should not use rosemary essential oil.

ROSEMARY

"Such strong roles I play, from following the bride in her bouquet to saying final farewells to those who cross over. In the cold I hide but am strong enough to break through the ice and be first to welcome the spring-time sun. I can be the quiet strength that carries you soothed through a bumpy day. All that is needed is your permission."

Energizing Foot Bath

For an energizing foot bath, fill a shallow basin with warm water. Sprinkle 2 fistfuls of rosemary sprigs (or 10 drops of rosemary essential oil) in the water, and soak your feet for 10 minutes. If you have Epsom salts, add 2 tablespoons. Visualize that you are gathering the fragmented parts of yourself—the part of you that lost your temper at work because you were scared of missing a deadline or frustrated after spending too long in traffic or lonely because of being misunderstood by your partner. It is when life is most difficult that we are called to the center, to the center of our being, the center of the world, to the stillness of the breath that unites all living beings. Open your heart and allow the peace that comes with forgiveness, letting go, and acceptance to find you. Breathe through all the craziness of your day, bringing calm and a sense of well-being to all the many aspects of you that are not separate, but the many faces of the diamond that is you. Connect with the faerie essence of rosemary and imagine the new and refreshed energy coursing through your body. And breathe.

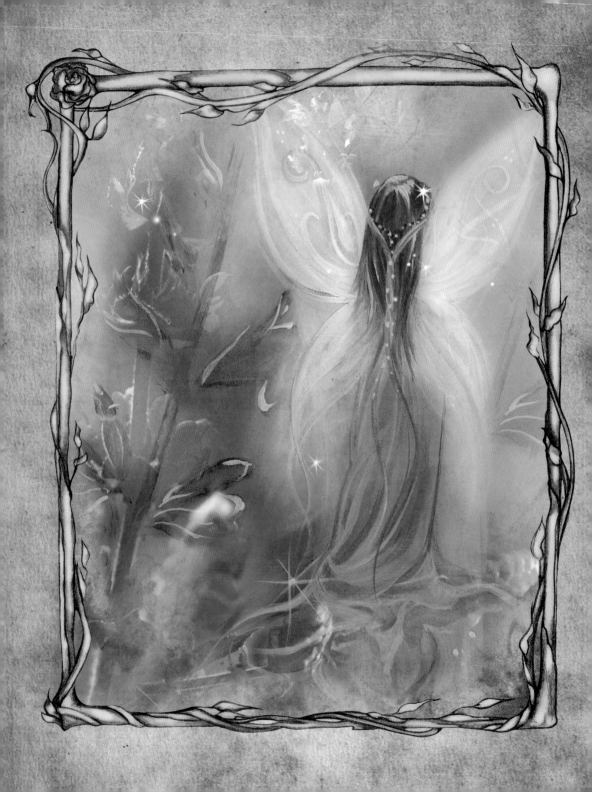

Sage

Salvia officinalis

Common Sage, Garden Sage, Smudge

PARTS USED: LEAVES, STEMS

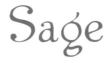

Sage originated from the island of Crete and generally grows about a foot or more high. The grayish green, softly hairy, oblong leaves are set in pairs on the stem. The flowers of garden sage, which blossom in August, appear in whorls of purple. All parts of the plant have a strong, scented odor and a warm, bitter, somewhat astringent taste, due to the volatile oil contained in the tissues. Sage prefers full sun and alkaline soil with little moisture.

Its botanical name, *salvia*, is derived from the Latin word *salvus*, meaning "healthy," and refers to the plant's curative powers, which have been known to treat stomach and intestinal ailments, menopausal symptoms, irregular menstrual bleeding, sore throats and gums, excessive sweating, restlessness, and kidney and urinary tract infections. It also stimulates the appetite, has a beneficial effect on the liver, and relieves indigestion. One legend says that the healing properties of sage come directly from the Virgin Mary.

In the tenth century, Moorish physicians believed that sage could extend life to the point of immortality. This belief sparked the medieval adage "Why should a man die while sage grows in his garden?" and the English proverb "He that would live foraye (forever) must eat sage in May." It was also believed that sage enhances one's prosperity and can ease grief, which is the reason it is sown in graveyards, particularly in France, where the belief originated.

Sage was introduced into China in the sixteenth century by Dutch explorers. Traditional Chinese Medicine uses sage to treat insomnia, depression, gastrointestinal complaints, mental illness, menstrual complaints, and mastitis. In Ayurvedic medicine, sage is used for the same complaints, but is also used to treat hemorrhoids, gonorrhea, vaginitis, and eye disorders.

Sage is used in many forms, including tea, vinegar, tincture, essential oil, and culinary spice. A sage leaf can be chewed and applied directly to a minor wound to staunch bleeding. You can rub a leaf over your teeth and tongue, like you would a toothbrush, to cool your mouth and freshen your breath. Sage tea can inhibit milk production in lactating women, reduce excessive sweating, stimulate appetite, and be used as a gargle for sore throats.

Sage is used in many natural beauty remedies and products, including hair rinses, facial packs for oily skin, and foot balms for problem feet. Sage carries warming qualities, and when 10 drops of the essential oil are combined with 15 drops of ginger essential oil, $^1/_2$ cup (113 milliliters) of wheat germ oil, and $^1/_2$ cup (113 milliliters) of jojoba oil, the combined oil provides relief for cold and damp feet.

White sage (*Salvia apiana* or *Salvia alpine*) is different than the sage variety used in the methods described above and is most often used in the form known as a smudge stick. A smudge stick is a bundle of dried white sage leaves burned for protection and purification of a space. White sage grows wild in mild climates. When gathering sage, be certain to make an offering to the plant, such as water or a piece of hair. This tradition has been employed by Native Americans for centuries, who will often fast prior to the gathering and sing during the harvest in respect of the sentient fae energy of the sage. Gathering and using white sage is in common use today by anyone wishing to clear an area of negative energy.

Sage invokes the deity Consus, the ruling god of councils. It seems probable from this connection that ancient people began using sage to purify and protect a room before a ritual. All ritual ceremonies are strongest when there is a consensus that binds together the collective desire of the community, i.e., for healing a sickness, gathering an abundant crop, promoting peace, etc.

Sage Herbal Vinegar

The fae energy of sage can produce calm when there is chaos, fulfillment where there is emptiness, and encouragement where there is depression. Sage accomplishes all this with the loving touch of Mother Mary. Nothing is impossible with sage at your side. This recipe brings together the healing energy of all the plants and serves to complement any salad dish.

INGREDIENTS

¹/₄ cup (55 grams) chopped sage leaves
¹/₄ cup (55 grams) chopped oregano leaves
¹/₄ cup (55 grams) chopped basil leaves
¹/₄ cup (55 grams) chopped marjoram leaves
I cup (250 milliliters) wine vinegar

Place the herbs in a glass pint jar and cover with wine vinegar. Shake well.

Yields I cup (250 milliliters)

SAGE

"Reach with me for the warmth of the sun. Let us dig our roots in deeply and draw from the knowledge of what we know in our hearts. Together we shall discover peace and community. Knowing what is within will show us what is real."

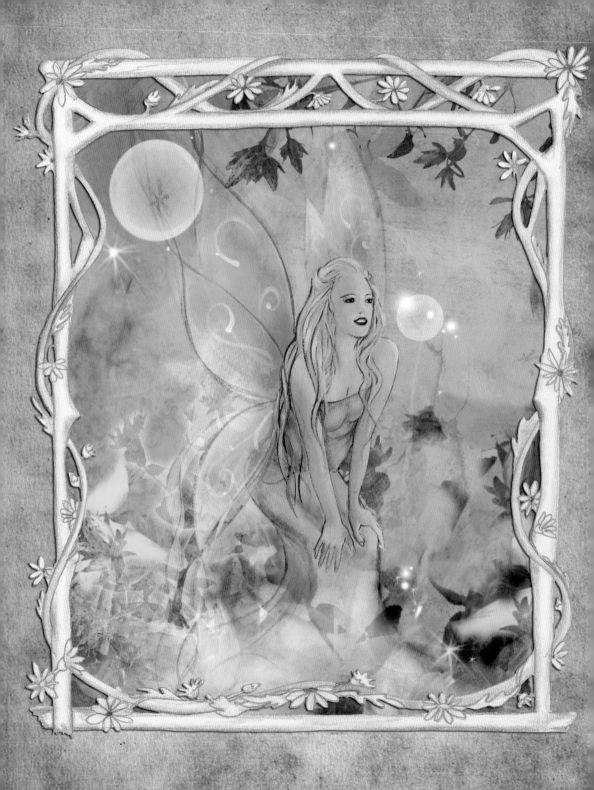

St. John's Wort

Hypericum perforatum

Herba Jon, Hyperisum, Klamath Weed, Raisin Rose,
St. Joan's Wort, Touch-and-Heal

PARTS USED: LEAVES, STEMS, FLOWERS

St. John's wort's leaves are frail and multiform with bright specks. The herb is recognized by the small, bright yellow, poppy-shaped flowers. It can reach a height of 2 to 3 feet. St. John's wort prefers sunny, warm locations, but will grow in partial shade. It likes well-drained soil, not too moist, with high humus content, preferring organic compost in the spring.

St. John's wort has a long history of being quite effective in healing wounds and is an effective nervine, with the added ability as an instant pain reliever. The herb derives its medicinal benefits from a high concentration of hypericin, a red pigment that exudes from its flowers, even when pinched. Inexplicably, St. John's wort grew in great abundance around old churches. In time, the red pigment was believed to represent the blood of St. John the Baptist and was used for protection, often in pomanders, since the Middle Ages.

Today, St. John's wort is commonly used to relieve fatigue, obsessive compulsive disorder, and depression, particularly seasonal affective disorder (SAD.) Its association with St. John is an interesting connection to SAD, given that this saint's feast day falls in the beginning of summer. The fae essence of St. John's wort simply makes you happy.

Touch-and-Heal Oil

ST. JOHNS' WORT

"What do you call beloved? I can see, can you? I'm looking ever so closely and think if I sprinkle just a bit of my sparkle in the right place, something beautiful would arise. Would you like to try? Shhhhh, just relax, let go, and believe."

The ingredients in this oil make it a practical remedy for relieving itchy or dry scabs and abrasions; reducing the appearance of scars; healing sprains, bruises, and burns; and soothing rough, chapped skin. This herb is an antispasmodic and an excellent remedy for muscle tension and back pain. The method of preparation makes it magickal! Based on an old Polish tradition, gather fresh St. John's wort on June 24, St. John's Day. Alternately, buy some St. John's wort on that day if fresh harvest is not possible. Also gather fresh or dried comfrey, peppermint, and lavender. How much of each? Polish ancestresses say, "Handfuls!"

In ancient times, Polish women of marriageable age would prepare an oil of St. John's wort each summer, and then compare their oils' appearances. Whoever had the "reddest" oil was expected to marry within the year. For information or visions about your beloved, drizzle a few drops of this oil into a bowl of water and gaze into it by candlelight. Remember, a beloved can also be a child, right livelihood, a home, travels, or anything you desire or love. Swirl your fingers in the water and oil and observe the patterns it makes on the surface of the water. Interpret according to your own symbolic understanding and intuition. This is a perfect project for a women's circle, garden club, or group of friends who want to make herbal magick together.

This ancient remedy works best when you follow your own internal wisdom. Use your own judgment, but typically, three parts St. John's wort are combined with two parts comfrey, and one part each peppermint and lavender, and then covered with oil. However, we have provided exact measurements in case this is your preference.

INGREDIENTS

2 cups (450 grams) dried St. John's wort flowers
1 cup (225 grams) dried comfrey leaves
1/2 cup (113 grams) dried peppermint leaves
1/2 cup (113 grams) dried lavender flowers
1 quart (1 liter) jojoba oil

Combine all the ingredients in a jar. Allow this herb-oil mixture to steep in its jar for one full moon cycle. Shake the jar, sing to it, dance around with it from time to time. If stuck for a song, then trace the outline of trees or plants, and allow the scale of your song to rise and fall with the contours of the foliage.

For extra potency, bury the jar out in your garden, allowing the power of the earth and fae magick to send its energy into the oil. Then excavate it at the appointed time. Heat the oil and herb mixture gently over a low flame, or in a double boiler, for 15 to 20 minutes. Allow to cool, strain out the herbs, and you have a great healing oil. For easier, tidier healing on the go, mix one part of this oil with one part solid coconut oil and half part molten beeswax. Mix well and allow to cool for a creamy, nourishing salve.

Yields approximately 1 liter, enough for eight 4-ounce (113-milliliter) jars

This recipe was donated by Rabbit, an ordained High Priestess and wandering magician, soothsayer, storyteller, and owner of the Sacred Well in Berkeley, California.

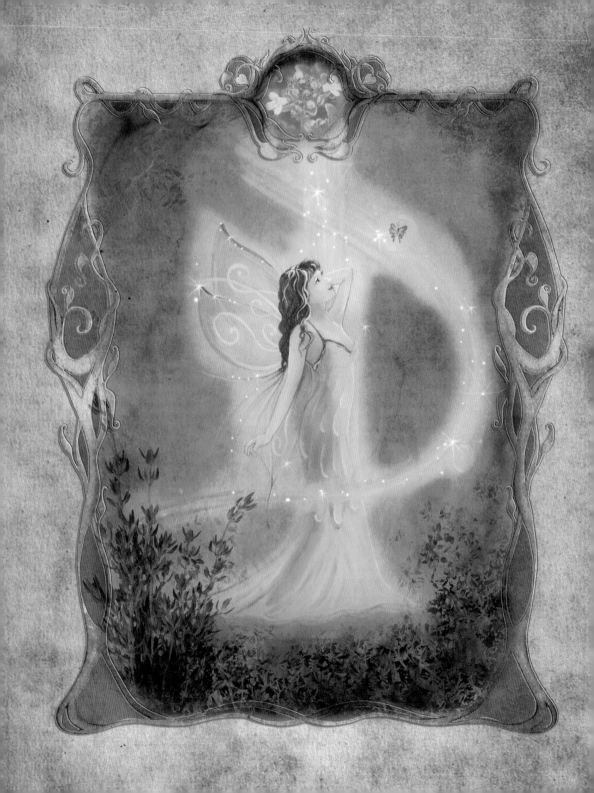

Thyme

Thymus vulgaris

Common Thyme, Garden Thyme

PARTS USED: FLOWERS, LEAVES

T he leaves of thyme are flat, dark, and highly aromatic. It has tiny pinkish flowers. Thyme grows wild on heaths and sunny banks. It prefers light, dry, well-drained soil and full to partial shade. It is recommended to cut off the shoots about 4 inches above the soil line shortly before the plant blooms in May or June. Bundle the herb together and hang the stems upside down in a dry, shaded place. You can use the herb as needed.

Thyme is a good source of iron and is used widely in culinary dishes. It is a basic ingredient in Arabian, Caribbean, French, Greek, Italian, Lebanese, Persian, Portuguese, Libyan, Spanish, Syrian, and Turkish cuisines.

This herb faerie essence confers tranquility, peace, security, and courage. Ancient Egyptians used thyme in embalming. The ancient Greeks used it in their baths and burnt it as incense in their temples, believing that thyme was a source of courage. It is possible that the word *thyme* is derived from the Greek word *thumus*, meaning "courage," however, it is also associated with the phrase "to make a burnt offering." As such, it is important to remember that the word *sacrifice* means to "make holy." Giving an offering or sacrifice to a deity represents the sacrosanct exchange of giving up something when you are asking to receive something new, more, or possibly improved. It is akin to the modern concept of paying it forward.

In the European Middle Ages, women would often give knights and warriors scarfs with embroidered sprigs of thyme. It was believed that the mere image of the herb would call upon the fae energy and bring valor and courage to the bearer. In this age, the herb was also placed beneath pillows to aid sleep and ward off nightmares, and today it is still used for this same purpose.

Thyme yields thymol, an essential oil, which is used as a disinfectant and in hair lotions. It is possible that thyme's ability to purify or cleanse aided its propensity to lend courage. Courage to clean a messy house? Perhaps. Two tablespoons of thyme essential oil mixed with 2 tablespoons salt and 2 tablespoons baking soda creates an excellent cutting-board disinfectant. Thyme is also believed to fortify the immune system with its warming qualities. Its strong antibacterial agents help fight the flu, colds, and even bronchitis. Combined with eucalyptus and lemon essential oils, it can be burned in an aromatherapy diffuser to protect against infection and help cleanse stale air. This would be an excellent warding-off winter chills combination. A couple drops of thyme essential oil added to $1/2$ cup (120 milliliters) of your favorite shampoo is believed to help prevent hair loss.

Many magickal folk use thyme to invoke faeries. According to the medieval point of view, the faeries were to be feared and avoided. The fae folk caused great mischief at a time of darkness and much fear. Some believe that due to the position of the earth in relation to the sun, there was limited refracted light. Medieval people could not perceive pastel colors. It was truly a dark and drab time. And yet, for those who were brave and able to face whatever the fae folk might bring, some people planted thyme as an invitation to the faeries. Thyme has been used to increase clairvoyance or clear seeing.

Thyme-for-Strength Bath Scrub

When you invoke the faeries with this plant, you will gain protection and the courage to see through your blind spots. Thyme is associated with Venus, who is represented by the Virgin. A virgin is not someone who is simply chaste and has not had sexual intercourse. The original meaning for a virgin is someone who has complete ownership of his or herself. A true virgin is a person who has inner strength to follow her true voice, listen to her innate wisdom, and follow her dreams. As you create and use this bath scrub, tap into your virginal self. Allow the fae energy of thyme to guide you back to the pure part of your being that is deeply in tune with your own rhythms, courage, and protection.

When you are in need of making connection with the wisdom and clarity of you, rub the bath scrub briskly onto damp skin before bathing, then rise off. Visualize a single flame burning at the center of your being. This light is pure and contains the essence that is your unique expression of the creative source. The entire universe is contained in this flame, and yet there is a particular way in which the flame moves and dances that is only captured by you. Celebrate in the individuality of the light that is you.

THYME

"As we spend our time together, you may enjoy my sensual aroma. As I entice you to dine and pull you into the circle of fae, I am also here to remind you to stay grounded. Don't lose your head or float away just yet!"

INGREDIENTS

3 cups (675 grams) coarse oatmeal
I cup (225 grams) dried thyme leaves
  and flowers
I cup (225 grams) dried scented rose petals
  or 5 drops rose-otto oil
Dried orange peel from 2 medium oranges

Working in small batches, grind the ingredients with a mortar and pestle. Work in a counterclockwise direction, imagining that you are willingly letting go of all that no longer serves you. Store in a cool dark place.

Yields 5 cups (1125 grams)

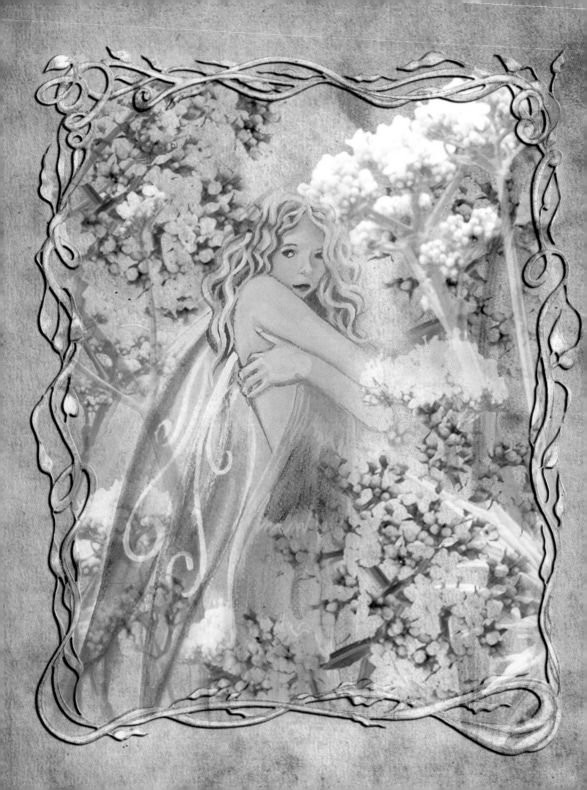

Valerian

Valeriana officinalis

All Heal, Amatilla, Capon's Tail, English Valerian, Garden Heliotrope,
Moon Root, Set Well, St. George's Herb, Vandal Root

PARTS USED: ROOTS

Valerian leaves are shiny and dark green. It is a perennial herb with branching stems that grow erect and sturdy, up to 5 feet tall. The plant has a crowning mass of white or rose-colored flowers, which bloom from June to September. Valerian prefers full sun and moist, humusy soil, and grows well in marshy thickets and on the borders of ditches and rivers. The plant is found throughout Europe and Northern Asia, and is common in England.

Valerian is best known for promoting a good night's sleep. Herbalists (and even some conventional medical practitioners) today cannot say enough about how sleep affects our general well-being. The herb's Latin name, *valeriana*, means "well-being," which points to the fact that everyone must rest. In today's society we often rush through things in an attempt to accumulate more—more experiences, more toys, more relationships. But without taking the time to absorb the information, the experiences have no real influence or effect.

Valerian faerie energy is root energy. It helps us feel grounded, find our center, and find comfort in our stillness. It is a Druid herb of consecration and purification and can be used in love and protection spells. In the Middle Ages the herb

VALERIAN

"Will you be my friend? Would you like to play with me in your dreams? I can guide you through your imagination and we can create anything you would like. I love to share and would be honored to share my gifts with you."

gained its nickname all heal for its ability to cure epilepsy—a frightening and misunderstood condition. In the aftermath of World War I, it was administered to shell-shocked soldiers.

Valerian's scent is usually abhorrent to most people, and many herbalists refer to the smell as reminiscent of a dirty sock. But after a while, many find the earthy aroma comforting thanks to the peace that comes with taking this herb. It is, in fact, the root herb for Valium, yet in a much gentler and natural way it induces sleep and well-being, all without addictive side effects or the serious aftereffects of other narcotics. Huzzah! It is also effective for easing anxiety, asthma, menstrual pain and cramps, and indigestion. It is most often taken in tea, tablet, and tincture form. The root can also be crushed and placed in "dream" sachets.

Recapitulation Dreaming

Lucid dreams, also known as conscious dreams, are dreams in which sleepers are aware that they are dreaming. When dreamers are lucid, they can actively participate in and often manipulate the imaginary experiences in the dream environment. Lucid dreaming is quite effective when you want to change a bad situation or change the direction of your life, but you don't know how.

Either tea or tincture of valerian will work for this meditation. You can choose to drink a cup of tea or take a dropperful of valerian tincture in 1 cup (250 milliliters) of water. Before going to bed, think about your situation. Cast around in your imagination for a simple item, such as a seashell, a bracelet, or a book. Sit quietly for a couple of minutes and ask the valerian to show you this special item in your dream. When you see your special item, you will awaken to the fact that you are dreaming and have the ability to manipulate the events of your dream to the most joyful conclusion. In this state, your logic cannot tell you what is possible. For in dreams, your world is illimitable.

The fae energy of valerian will show you that simple item and the entire dream message will come flooding back to you. The faeries will bless you with visions of how to create peace and harmony in a stressful situation or right direction, whatever it is you need.

Sometimes it is necessary to repeat this process as you become more and more comfortable with lucid dreaming. Keep at it. The visions will come.

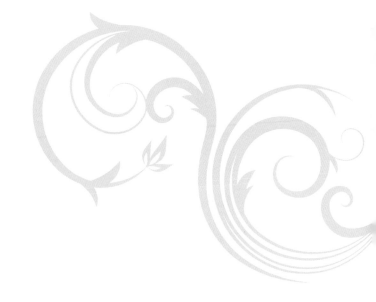

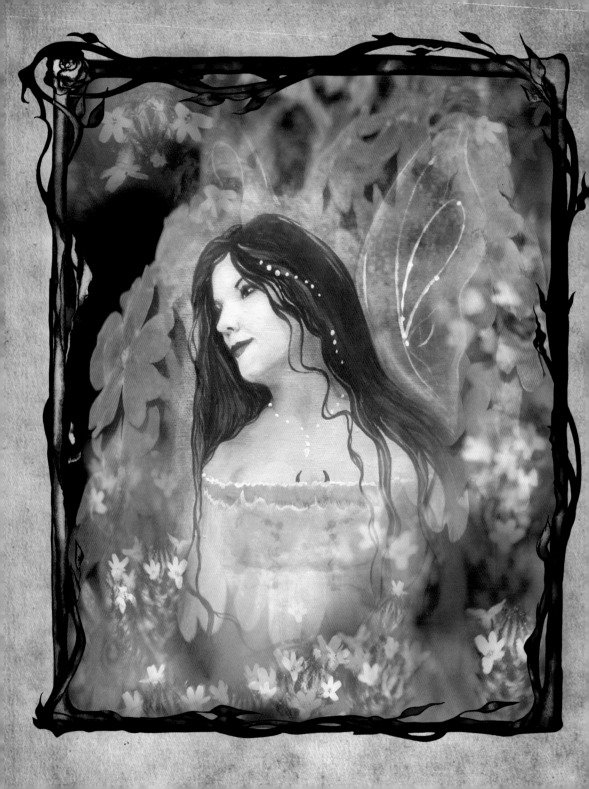

Vervain

Verbena officinalis

Blue Vervain, Enchanter's Plant, Herb of Grace, Herb-of-the-Cross,
Juno's Tears, Pigeon's Grass, Simpler's Joy, Tears of Isis

PARTS USED: LEAVES, FLOWERS, STEMS

Vervain flowers are small, with five petals, are borne in dense spikes and come in shades of blue, white, pink, or purple. It prefers full sun and moderately fertile, well-drained, but moisture-retentive soil.

Vervain is a strengthening tonic and as a tea stimulates the appetite and has a calming effect, making it a successful herb to treat irritable bowel syndrome, nervous indigestion, and colitis. It is also used as a mild natural tranquilizer and is often used to treat anxiety, particularly when linked to menstrual, menopausal, digestive, and bronchial problems. Vervain has been used to treat abdominal pain, nausea, insomnia, restlessness, nerve pain, digestive problems, skin irritations, colds, and headaches. A compress of the tea will alleviate minor wounds, eczema, and hemorrhoids, whereas a compress soaked in a cooling vinegar-vervain decoction can ease joint pain.

Vervain is used to attract prosperity. A simple ritual includes taking a handful of dried vervain and sprinkling it over your home. Dance

VERVAIN

"Come sit with me a spell and let's talk of love, true, undying, and gentle and yet so strong. It is immortal."

over the herbs, envisioning the abundance that is coming your way. Sweep the herb in a clockwise circle to symbolize the gathering of your wealth. Offer the vervain as compost to a tree or plant in the north—the direction of grounding.

According to Egyptian lore, vervain originated from the tears of Isis as she wept for her husband Osiris. It was a very important herb to the Roman god Jupiter and was at a special place on his altar. During the Middle Ages, it was believed to ward off the plague. It was considered an Herb of Immortality among the Druids and was worn in amulets as protection. It is associated with many deities, including Aradia, Cerridwen, Diana, Mars, and Thor.

Do not take vervain during pregnancy, because it induces uterine contractions.

Vervain Love Incense

The herb is often gathered at Midsummer, also known as Summer Solstice or Litha, a very active time for fae energy. Just think about all the buzzing bees, active energy, and tingly sensations of summer, when life is at its most juicy and succulent. The fae are awake because the garden is awake. Midsummer is a time to recognize that even though the sun is at its zenith, from this point forward the days will grow shorter, the nights longer. It is a celebration of life at its most abundant and yet a reckoning with the fact that light must give way to night in the ever-turning cycle of life. In this way, we see the faerie essence of this plant and its connection to immortality. The theme also runs through the story of Isis and her love for Osiris, whom she brought back from the dead through her determination to believe in true, everlasting love. This incense will draw love to you of the kind that cannot be tarnished, but survives through mutual respect and calm understanding of each other's individuality.

INGREDIENTS

3 tablespoons dried vervain flowers
3 tablespoons dried rose petals
3 tablespoons ground cinnamon

Place all the herbs in a mortar and pestle and grind them into a powder in a clockwise direction. While you are doing this, think about the attributes you want your
love to have: attentive, passionate, communicative, generous. Do you want a playmate?
An equal? A confidant? Be as precise about the soul and light of the person, without
attributing physical qualities. Light a piece of charcoal. When the charcoal turns
white, sprinkle the incense on top and chant or say:

"By these three herbs I call love to me
To settle in my life ever so calmly.
I will trust, however, the one who comes to me
This I make true, Three Times Three Times Three."

Yields just over ¼ cup (65 grams)

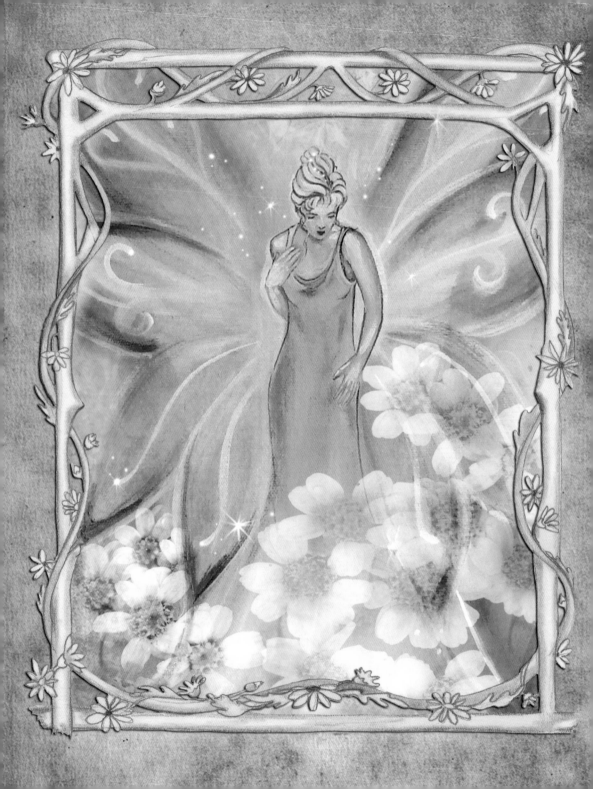

Yarrow

Achillea millefolium

Bloodwort, Devil's Plaything, Hundred-Leaved Grass,
Knight's Milfoil, Milfoil, Nosebleed, Old Man's Pepper,
Seven Year's Lore, Soldier's Woundwort, Thousand-Heal

PARTS USED: FLOWERS, LEAVES, STEMS

The yarrow stem is angular and rough, the leaves alternate, 3 to 4 inches long and 1 inch broad, and have a feathery appearance. Its flowers appear from June to September, and are white or pale lilac, looking like minute daisies. The whole plant is more or less hairy, with white, silky appressed hairs. Yarrow is a perennial ground cover that likes moderately rich, well-drained soil and full sun. It does not require a lot of watering, unless in a pot.

Yarrow is believed to have derived its Latin name, *Achillea millefolium*, from the Greek lore that the warrior Achilles used yarrow to treat his battle wounds during the Trojan War. The plant has been used for centuries to heal wounds and to stem bleeding. It can decrease internal hemorrhaging and is anti-inflammatory and anti-microbial. It is used as a tea, a tincture, an essential oil, and an ingredient in natural beauty products. Native Americans used yarrow to take the throbbing pain out of bee stings, ease childbirth, treat breast abscesses, and expel the placental afterbirth. In esoteric practices, yarrow is used to attract love, increase clairvoyance, and provide protection.

Yarrow tea helps stomach complaints and poor digestion, improves circulation, strengthens weak veins, eases menstrual bleeding, and stems coughing. Yarrow essential oil has astringent, antibacterial, and some anti-inflammatory properties. Mix 4 to 6 drops of yarrow oil with cocoa butter to make a lotion that can help reduce stretch marks and varicose veins. For relief from acne, place 3 drops each of yarrow essential oil and bergamot essential oil in a bowl of steaming water. Lean over the bowl with a towel draped over your head. Allow the vapors to cleanse your pores for as long as possible. Yarrow poultices are used for muscle and joint pain as well as varicose veins and to draw out mild poisons.

Yarrow Meditation

In China, yarrow embodies the perfect union between the yin, or female, with its downy soft flowers, and yang, or male, with its erect stems. The essential oil brings balance to these opposing energies in the emotional body. If you see the first blossom in a yarrow patch, it is customary that you get to make a wish.

YARROW

"I am the last to meet you on this journey. I am the healing touch at the end of battle. The gentle end to a stress-filled day. With a rested mind and quiet soul I say hello and farewell. The perfect balance. But first, follow me into meditation so you may know me better."

We are mostly in action, always doing, producing, making, etc. But in meditation, we can begin to equalize the yang energy with the resting energy of yin. For this meditation, you will be creating a balance between the yin energy as symbolized by water or earth, which is considered the receptive, feminine force, and yang energy, as symbolized by fire or wind, which is the creative, masculine opposite of yin. While opposites, they are not absolutes—nothing can exist without each, and neither is superior to the other. You must find the right balance of yin and yang in your own life. You can make your own yarrow-infused oil or use yarrow essential oil. To make your own oil, fill a jar with yarrow flowers and leaves and cover with grapeseed oil and allow to sit for at least 2 weeks. Drain out the oil and discard the herb. Place 3 or 4 drops of yarrow essential oil on a diffuser or place infused oil on your pulse points at the wrist and neck and sit still.

Take a deep breath. Close your eyes. Listen to the sounds as they come to you: traffic, birds, voices out on the street. Allow them to be part of the world. Listen to the sounds within your body: your breathing, heartbeat. Turn all those sounds into one joined sound, like the sound of the ocean. Imagine yourself floating in this ocean, and as you breathe, allow yourself to sink further into the sea with each breath, deeper into your own being, deeper than your identity or story, deep into the oneness. Take a moment and feel centered.

In this ocean of being there is everything you need: health, serenity, and love. Take what you need most—peace of mind, unconditional love, physical health, or more patience and understanding. Don't be worried about choosing the wrong thing, because you can come back here any time and get anything else you desire. Imagine that the thing you need most is captured in a glowing ball of light that enters your being through your heart. Breathe in deeply, and take that good from the pure energy within you. It is now part of you, linked to who you are in the very depth of your soul.

As you slowly exhale, allow yourself to rise back to the physical world. Go slowly. Take a moment to regain awareness of your body, your arms, your shoulders, your legs, and your feet. Listen to the sounds of your breathing, and then the sounds outside of your body. Come back to the world. When you're ready, open your eyes.

CONCLUSION

A Love for All Living Things

Many of us were not brought up to believe spirituality or connection to the Divine could be found in nature—rather, we were led to believe that our relationship with the sacred was found indoors, in a church, synagogue, or temple, often requiring the help or translation of another more "qualified" individual. However, for many of us, particularly those reading this book, we discovered at an early age a deep calling to be close to nature and found more wonder and peace in the enfoldment of wildlife than we did in religious tomes or stained glass depictions. Whether we were talking to bees or hugging trees, or sitting all day on a grassy hill watching the wind make tree branches sway or snow fall gently, or smelling the dampness of early morning dew on flowers or wheat, or staying out way past the time when the streetlamps went on just to feel the cool night air and watch the twinkling of the first stars or the spectacular green flash at sunset, we *had* to be outside. It wasn't merely a desire; it was an intrinsic need that filled us with immense joy and pure exuberance. We were simply giddy to watch a spider spin her web or hummingbirds chase each other. We danced with delight when the crocuses or tulips first poked through the earth or when the time came to harvest the vegetables.

This deep connection with the heartbeat that radiates through all life is known as biophilia, or a love for all living things. The term *biophilia* was popularized and explored extensively by the conservationist, Father of Sociobiology, and two-time Pulitzer Prize winner E. O. Wilson in his *Biophilia Hypothesis*, which states that humans have a predisposition to be close to nature—as seen, for example, with our tendency to have pets, household plants, or gardens. This intrinsic need arose from our biological evolution and thousands of years as hunter-gatherers, so that in our DNA and the psyche we are most content when we are intimately tied to nature, wildlife, wildness, and cyclical seasons. It is the purpose of this book to support you in reestablishing or deepening that affiliation with nature by introducing you to thirty-three, easy-to-find herbs.

Every journey begins with a single step. We believe that developing a loving bond with herbs found in your garden can begin the exciting and fulfilling adventure back to an unshakable and secure connection to the core of all life. A loving bond with nature is at the center of green magick. Our ancestors knew that as long as they took care of Mother Earth, She would take care of them. The time has come to take better care of earth—our home.

"Thank you for allowing us to show you more of ourselves. It's been a beautiful experience, learning about one another, a most sacred dance. Thank you for letting us in. Now that you recognize us you can invite us back at any time. Whether through our aromatic scents, beautiful blossoms, or spicy culinary adventures, we know you will see more than ever imagined before. The relationships we hope to forge with you carry the possibility to keep the magick alive not only in us, but in you as well. The only ingredient left for you to add is to *believe*."

Index